BRAND NEW NURSE

SURVIVING YOUR FIRST DAY ON THE JOB

DAVE DOVELL, RN

Brand New Nurse: Surviving Your First Day on the Job

Copyright © 2022 Dave Dovell

Forward written by Anne Llewellyn

Revised by Johnny Carroll

All rights reserved.

ISBN: 9798818106014

Contact: thenewRNblog@gmail.com

All rights reserved.

This book or parts thereof may not be reproduced in any form, stored in any retrieval system, or transmitted in any form by any means—electronic, mechanical, photocopy, recording, or otherwise—without prior written permission of the publisher, except as provided by United States of America copyright law.

Disclaimer: The information in this book is in no way intended to replace guidelines, protocols, or policies put in place by healthcare institutions. Always practice within your scope of practice and in accordance with your facility's guidelines. This book is intended for informational and entertainment purposes only and is not intended to provide instruction for the treatment of disease or injury.

BRAND NEW NURSE

SURVIVING YOUR FIRST DAY ON THE JOB

DAVE DOVELL, RN

DEDICATION

This book is dedicated to my fellow nurse, former study partner and now loving wife Marissa, my amazing son Noah, my mom Patty, dad Tony, and sister Jen for always supporting me, and my best friend Jon Crosier who is the reason I became a nurse in the first place.

TABLE OF CONTENTS

Forward

Preface

Introduction: *Getting Past those New Nurse Jitters*..1

Gearing Up for Your First Day..5

Doing Your Homework..19

Your First Hours on the Job..23

Get Yourself Organized..29

The Night Shift..39

Focus on the Important Stuff..49

Meet Your Preceptor..61

Building Relationships..67

Establishing Your Reputation..83

Communicating with Your Colleagues..99

Handling the Emotions..105

Conclusion: *A Sigh of Relief and a Nice Ride Home*......123

Meet the Contributors..126

71 Quick & Awesome Nursing Tips..128

FORWARD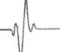

Forward by Anne Llewellyn, MS, BHSA, RN, CCM, CRRN, CMGT-BC, CM Fellow

As I retire from active practice and you enter the exciting nursing profession, I welcome you and wish you the best. A common saying fits our roles: "If you love what you do, you will never work a day in your life."

Nursing is the best job I have ever had - but I did not look at it as a job; I looked at it as a profession. It was the one job where I knew I was making a difference. I was an instrumental member of the healthcare team. Because of my training, I could help those who were sick, lonely, afraid, and in many cases facing the biggest challenge of their lives.

I am a nurse of over 40 years who has worked in various settings in two states. I became a nurse because I wanted something interesting and exciting. I entered as a Practical Nurse, then after a few years, gained my Registered Nurse license. I worked for several years as a critical care nurse in the emergency department and the Respiratory Intensive Care Unit. I saw the best and the worst of human beings and was surrounded by the best of those who made up the broad healthcare team. I then moved into Risk Management, where I saw another side of the healthcare system and learned how to react to medical errors and challenges caused by mistakes and challenges of our complex healthcare system. My subsequent two roles have

DAVE DOVELL, RN

been case management and patient/health advocacy. These have been important roles in which I have learned a great deal about what it means to be a patient. Navigating the healthcare system is not easy, especially when you are sick, in pain, or frail due to age or medical conditions.

I felt my role as a nurse in whatever role I played, as needed, was influential and respected. I helped people in need and at the lowest moments in their lives with respect and empathy. I helped people get back on their feet after a catastrophic injury and do things they never thought they would do because they had the tools they needed. I was able to do this as I was a nurse, a member of a team that included the patient, their family, physicians, other nurses, therapists, the employer, and the community. As a nurse, I learned how to understand the system so I could break down barriers and help people get the care they needed.

When I moved into Case Management and Patient/Health Advocacy, I learned how to advocate for my patients and their families when many said no. I worked with the patient and their family and helped them set realistic expectations and understand how important it was for them to have a voice in their care. Today, it is essential to encourage people to be active members and make sure their goals are met, and they get the care they want.

As an experienced nurse, I used my voice to make changes to benefit my patients and the team I worked with. I do not settle for the status quo, and I hope you don't.

I learned from foodservice carriers, the housekeeping staff, and up the chain. I also discovered all healthcare team members from my patients and their families. Every team member has a role, and as they say, we are better when we work together. Never dismiss a comment you might get from the housekeeper about a patient or the person who delivers meals. They have insights into our patients that can be valuable.

I learned that a 'thank you' from my patient and their families was worth more than I was being paid, as it helped me know that I had made a difference in their lives.

I hope you enjoy this book: *Brand New Nurse: Surviving your First Day on the Job.* It is an essential resource for every nurse entering the nursing profession and those who are veterans that will help them remember what our role is and the vital role each nurse plays in today's broad and complex healthcare system. I thank Dave Dovell for writing this book.

I wish you the best of luck for those new to the profession. Your role is essential. You have the basics to do this job, and you will gain confidence every day! Best of luck and remember you are an indispensable member of the healthcare team.

Anne Llewellyn, MS, BHSA, RN, CCM, CRRN, CMGT-BC, CM Fellow

DAVE DOVELL, RN

Anne is a registered nurse with over forty-three years of experience in critical care, risk management, case management, patient advocacy, and healthcare education, including training and development. Anne speaks and writes frequently on topics for consumers, caregivers, and all healthcare team members, so we can improve each person's healthcare experience. Follow her in her weekly Blog, Nurses Advocate, where she shares stories and events to help people be better prepared when they enter the healthcare system.

https://nursesadvocates.com

PREFACE

You studied for countless hours. You missed birthday parties, you weren't there to help move your friend across town, and sometimes your friends didn't even hear from you for weeks. But you were a nursing student embarking on the journey of a lifetime. Whatever jobs or careers you had before nursing school didn't seem to matter because you were learning to become a nurse. Each quiz, test, and practical mattered. Every clinical. Every care plan. Each concept that went over your head had to be relearned, studied, and understood because you weren't learning how to do accounting or how to prepare a recipe; you were learning to save lives.

The studying didn't end when you graduated. Your family couldn't wait to start seeing you at holidays and events again, but you jumped right back into your textbooks to prepare for the NCLEX. The months of preparation paid off and it seemed like forever before you learned that you had passed and officially became an RN. At that point, you wanted to sit back and relax. But a nursing license won't pay your bills unless you land a nursing job which, remarkably, you have done!

Is the stress over? Is the anxiety gone? Have you finally reached Easy Street?! Well, it's 2 o'clock in the morning. Your scrubs are laid out for your first day tomorrow, your fancy new nurse clogs are waiting by your front door, and you've already attached about 3 pounds of badge buddies to your zippy little badge holder. It *looks* like you are prepared for your very first shift as a registered nurse...but how do you *feel*?

It is completely normal to be anxious, excited, nervous, apprehensive...a million different feelings...before starting your first nursing job. After all, it all comes down to this moment! Tomorrow marks the first day of what will most likely be a long and rewarding career making a big difference in the lives of countless patients. I hope this book will help settle your nerves, prepare you for what your first day will bring, and reassure you that you are absolutely where you are supposed to be right now.

The over 4 million nurses in the United States represent over 4 million "very first days." Each nurse working in this world has been precisely where you are now and has made it through their orientations successfully. You are probably more awesome than a bunch of those other nurses, so what are you worried about? Maybe you're stressed that you won't arrive at work prepared. Or maybe interacting with all new colleagues is freaking you out a bit. Is it simply that you won't know where the bathroom is on your first day 'cause that's a real thing, too!

Hopefully, you're reading this a bit earlier than the night before your first shift and this book will make your transition from the "civilian" world to the world of nursing a smooth one. If it truly is 2 am and you've picked this book up for the first time simply because you've tried everything else to sleep but you can't get your tummy to settle down and your brain to switch off, that's okay too. I can't promise you won't be tired tomorrow, but I am confident that YOU will be more confident. Through the advice I have collected from both my own experiences and the combined experience of my many colleagues and contributors, you can and will walk into your first nursing shift confident, prepared, and ready to make a difference.

—

Speaking of my experience, you might be wondering what gives me the authority to guide you through the first day of your career. Allow me to introduce myself: I'm Dave and it was just a few short years ago that I was sitting right where you are. My journey started back in 2012. I had graduated from Rutgers University with a Bachelor's in History and a state teacher's license, but I found my dream teaching job always got scooped up by a principal's daughter, gym teacher's niece, or department head's husband. I had some free time, so I signed up with my local fire department to volunteer. On my first day, they asked if I'd like to be an EMT or firefighter. I wasn't sure, so the Captain asked if I wanted to respond to 900 calls a year or 5,000. I said I didn't mind running my butt off so off to the EMT academy he sent me.

I worked on an ambulance responding to 911 calls, everything from heart attacks to house fires, for several years. I became a crew chief, then a mentor where I would take other new EMT recruits under my wing and train them until they became certified. I loved every second of my time in emergency services but never considered it a career until my best friend passed away.

My buddy Jon was like the brother I never had. One day at the age of 29, he just didn't feel well. He was shortly thereafter diagnosed with leukemia. He fought like hell and, at one point, he even thought he beat his cancer. But it came back after a few months and he never made it out of the hospital again. I spent countless hours in his hospital room chatting with him, watching Phillies games, stealing Ensure shakes, and just hanging out. It was his nurses that inspired me to become an RN myself.

These nurses were EXPERTS. The way they explained his lab tests, his procedures, and his plan of care. They titrated his medications on the fly and went so far out of their way to make his last months on this planet comfortable. I was in awe. Nursing wasn't just about handing out pills and bedpans...it was about becoming an *expert* in making a difference. I decided I wanted to be that for other people and immediately signed up for nursing school. And got wait-listed.

Bullshit, I know. The silver lining: I was the VERY FIRST name on the waitlist. So when someone named Ira Sponsible didn't pay her program deposit on time, I got the call and was in for the fall semester! During school, I landed a job working in a busy ER as a tech. That job taught me every bit as much as my nursing labs did and, by the time I began clinicals, I was already quite comfortable with bedside care.

I studied harder than I ever had before. I immersed myself in nursing and started knocking down one class at a time until I had achieved my degree, blasted through the NCLEX, and nailed down my first nursing job. What a whirlwind of a few years.

I was hired on a cardiac stepdown unit at a specialty hospital. The patient load was heavy, acuity was high, but the people there were incredibly supportive and made my orientation a pleasure. Note I didn't say it was *easy*. But with the help of my preceptor, Lauren, some great nurses like John and Wanda, and my incredibly knowledgeable then-girlfriend/now-wife Marissa, I made it through.

So, just a few years later, I'm here to guide you through your first days as a brand new nurse (and it's still fresh in my mind!). I'm now a preceptor at my hospital and I take new nurses like you under my wing and show them the ropes. I believe and hope you will benefit from my victories, my mistakes, and all the tips and tricks that I picked up during my first years in what I can't wait to live out as an incredibly rewarding and interesting fun career.

Some advice from my contributors for your first day:

⚕ "Start by doing a lot more listening than talking." Michelle Lasota, RN

⚕ "Remember, you've already passed your NCLEX so you have what you need to be where you are." Wanda Goodmond, RN

⚕ "Be on time, or even a bit early." Patty Stark, RN

⚕ "Take notice of everybody's routine." Ray Lawton, RN

⚕ "Take it day by day. Don't be too hard on yourself; everyone was a new grad at some point." Tori Meskin, BSN, RN-NIC

⚕ "Be confident and love your patients, after all, that is what we are here for." John Davis, RN

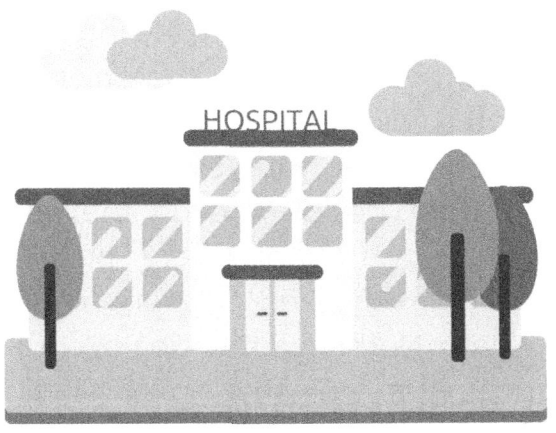

Introduction

Shaking off Those New Nurse Jitters

You have faced some challenging "firsts" in your life, from your first day of school to your first kiss, your first day with a driver's license, or the first day of college. Each of these firsts probably came with its own form of anxiety, nerves, and fear of the unknown. While your mind may have raced in the moments leading up to that first kiss or the first time you stepped foot in a nursing class, the pressure you felt did not come close to how you're feeling now.

As you turned onto the main hospital drive, you followed signs for "Employee Parking." Everything you need for your first day is sitting right beside you on the passenger seat; you know it's all there because you checked and rechecked at every red light on the way here. Nothing left to do now but switch off your car, grab your snazzy new nursing bag, and stroll into your brand new career.

As you swipe your badge and the staff entrance door opens, some of the nerves seem to disappear. You remember that, unlike millions of nurses before you who have crossed the threshold into their first shift, you are not alone. Nope, you've got a friend in your corner who can tell you what to expect, guide you through your first days of orientation, and remind you just how awesome you are. That friend is me.

Because I'm your friend, your first day is off to a smooth start. You remember reading about all the stuff to bring with you and your nursing bag has been packed for two days. You got a great night's sleep so you could show up on Day One bright-eyed and bushy-tailed. Hell, you even arrived 15 minutes early because you accounted for traffic, weather, animal crossings, and drawbridge openings. Look at you being an overachiever!

Joking aside, you have NOTHING to worry about. Your first day will be packed with new faces, names, paperwork, guidelines, protocols, logins, and passwords. You can't be expected to remember it all, so write down as much as you can, keep a smile on your face, and stay excited. You worked incredibly hard to be here and have all the book knowledge to be successful. Pay attention and take it all in today. You're only the *new* nurse once, so enjoy it and try to have fun.

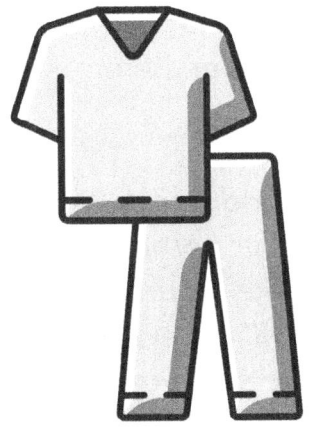

Gearing Up for Your First Day

The Shopping Spree Years in the Making

Gearing up for your first day as a Registered Nurse can be the most fun part of starting your new job. You've worked extremely hard to get to this point and it's completely normal to want to reward yourself. The economy scrubs, stethoscope, and shoes you picked up for nursing school may be wearing out and you're excited to start upgrading, so let's get into the top gear to consider before starting your first day as a nurse.

> *Wanda Goodmond, RN says "Your first day starts at home so look in the mirror. You look like a nurse. Your shoes and uniform will tell everyone you're a nurse. Now make sure you have your equipment: your pens (more than one), penlight, scissors, calipers, and stethoscope. Now breathe…"*

Scrubs

The most noticeable and one of the most important items you'll want to pick up are new scrubs. The key factors in choosing scrubs are fit and durability. You will live in these scrubs for long shifts, sometimes over 14 hours at a time, all the while you'll be moving, squatting, lifting, pushing, and pulling. Your scrubs must be able to move with you and work as hard as you are.

There are some great scrubs out there that have great fabric and features but won't break the bank. Shop around and be patient in your hunt for the perfect scrubs. You may have to purchase one pair to wear for a while to determine if you want more of the same. I always look for scrubs that have stretch to them and a nice synthetic fabric that won't fade after a few dozen rounds through the laundry. Pocket placement is something else to consider, especially if you're like me and you MUST have cargo pockets on the pants.

You'll often be tempted by unique prints and eclectic new colors as scrub companies strive to set themselves apart. Depending on your facility, you may have strict guidelines as to what colors and prints you are permitted to wear; make sure you find this out before shopping. For your first day, I would recommend not pushing the envelope with your scrub fashion choices. You will want to be taken seriously and wearing a set of professional-looking scrubs can play a large role in that first impression.

Shoes

Not enough can be said about choosing high-quality footwear when working as a nurse. Depending on your position and facility, you may spend over 12 hours a day on your feet and your shoes will be the deciding factor between a good day and a painful one. Many schools of thought exist regarding the perfect nursing shoe, ranging from clogs to Crocs, trail runners to cross-trainers. The choice you make will be based on your preferences and may change over time. I'll briefly go over a few options and weigh the pros and cons of each.

Clogs

Pros: Durable, easy on and off, good mechanical protection, great liquid protection.
Cons: Comfort levels vary, difficult to move quickly or walk backward when moving equipment or patients.

Crocs

Pros: Durable, easy on and off, good liquid protection (as long as they aren't the "holey" kind!), comfortable for most, affordable
Cons: You can't use aftermarket insoles to customize comfort, unprofessional looking, also can be difficult moving quickly or walking backward (yes, even in 4x4 sport mode).

Trail Runners

Pros: One of my favorites, I like the arch support, extra protection in the toe box, and rugged outsoles. Great mechanical protection and great liquid protection if waterproof.

Cons: Not all nurses like lace-up shoes for work because the laces can drag on the ground and get quite disgusting. Also, can't kick feet out easily to let 'em breathe during breaks.

Running/Cross Training Sneakers

Pros: Lightweight, easy to find a custom fit, moderate mechanical protection, moderate liquid protection if waterproofing spray is used, breathable, plenty of "laceless" options available.

Cons: Not as durable, sometimes sneakers will wear out within 3-6 months of heavy wear at work. Depending on the sneaker, less protection than other options out there for your feet. Still, I tend to choose either sneakers or trail runners over the others for comfort and mobility.

Socks

If no one has preached the importance of compression socks to you yet, you may want to consider finding better nurse friends. Just like the anti-embolic stockings you were taught to put on all your patients in nursing school, compression socks will become a mainstay in your daily wardrobe. They help prevent swelling in your feet, ankles, and calves. Your legs will be less fatigued after a long shift of standing and/or running around. Plus there are so many varieties of compression socks available specifically for nurses, it is a fun way to express yourself without going nuts with the rest of your uniform.

Backpack

This may be something you already have and don't need to purchase, but a good high-quality backpack is essential to use as a work bag. I like a backpack rather than a shoulder bag, satchel, or tote for several reasons. The two-strap carry is easier on your back after a long day. You'll want plenty of space in the bag for bulkier items like an extra set of scrubs. I also like that many backpacks have an "admin pocket" with slots for pens and small items; it makes it much easier to keep your bag organized. Ladies, I've seen some of your over-the-shoulder bags for work and how everything is just tossed in…I could never do it.

In your bag, you'll want to keep an extra set of scrubs in case things at work get a little too messy, pens, snacks, water bottles, liquid bandage for annoying knicks and cuts on your hands, and any personal items you may need throughout the shift.

Stethoscope

Your need for the world's greatest stethoscope may vary based on the type of nursing you will be doing. The price difference between decent stethoscopes and great ones is drastic, so it may be a good idea to start small and upgrade once you figure out exactly what you'll need. I work in cardiology and frequently perform an in-depth assessment of the heart and lung sounds, therefore I need a high-end stethoscope. You may not need to make this sort of investment if you work in a different area of nursing such as psych or orthopedics.

Something nurses always look forward to after getting their nursing license is that first big birthday or holiday afterward when your family can flood you with nursing gifts! This is a good opportunity to upgrade your stethoscope and it gives your family a chance to give you a gift you will actually use and not just another "cute enough to stop your heart" T-shirt.

Shears

There are two kinds of nurses in every hospital. Those who carry trauma shears on them at all times and those who borrow trauma shears on a routine basis. I began carrying shears on me when I worked as an EMT for obvious reasons. I continued to carry them when I started as an ER technician and discovered how many uses a solid pair of shears could have: everything from cutting gauze and dressings, opening tricky medications and packages, performing small repairs on equipment, and more.

Now, on my cardiology unit, I don't see trauma patients anymore but I still use my shears daily. As far as I'm concerned, there are three classes of trauma shears, ranging in price and quality. I avoid the cheapos personally but for many nurses, they work just fine. I carried Leatherman Raptors with me on the ambulance and loved them. They are too heavy for my scrub pants, so now they live clipped to the trauma bag in my truck. My all-time favorite shears for hospital use are the North American

Rescue Trauma Shears, as they are affordable, robust, and have nice features like rubberized handles and an oxygen wrench. Here are the pros and cons of each class of trauma shears:

Cheapos

Pros: cheap, cost around $1-2. No depression if they are lost or get messed up. Good for light duty like dressings, tape, packages.
Cons: Not durable, if used for any heavy cutting will often need replacement.

Midrange

Pros: Affordable, usually $8-15, much higher quality than cheapos. Good for all cutting. Lightweight.
Cons: May not have all the fanciness of top range shears, you'll be sadder if they get lost.

Top Range
(we're talking about Leatherman Raptor Shears here)

Pros: Full-featured, extremely durable, gear junkies will break their necks trying to sneak a peek at your Raptors.

Cons: Too heavy to wear with scrub pants and pricey enough that you definitely don't want to lose them.

Clipboard

A folding clipboard to be exact. Carrying a clipboard has completely changed how I organize my day as a nurse. I strongly recommend using one, as it's the best way to keep your report sheets, daily notes, and to-do lists all in one place. I will even take my clipboard with me when I shop for scrubs to ensure it will fit in my cargo pocket. No matter where I am, that little clipboard ensures I have all of my assessment data with me, important lab values, updated plans of care, and more. If I lost my clipboard tomorrow, I would immediately go get a new one…that's how you know a piece of gear is valuable to you.

> *Ray Lawton, RN says "Remember, less is more. As you start out, take notice of what you use and what you actually need throughout your shift. Keep the other stuff in a designated gear bag. And always keep a copy of your own personal report sheet!"*

Writing tools

This all comes down to preference. My family showered me with all sorts of gifts when I was about to start my first shift and this included some writing tools. I always have a decent black pen for my everyday writing. I also keep a 4-color pen on me which I use to organize my report sheets. Every nurse has a unique method for organizing report sheets based on their needs; I like to color-code my notes based on when the information is obtained. For instance, black writing is for my initial report notes on the patient, blue is for any updates that happen during the shift, green is used for future shift updates if I have the same patient for longer than a day, and red is a critical item.

I also like having a dry erase marker on me so I can update my patients' boards. Highlighters are helpful for report sheets but also when reviewing discharge information with patients. Lastly, I like keeping a small Sharpie around for labeling items.

Water bottle

I am guilty of not practicing what I preach here, but staying hydrated during your shift is incredibly important. The chips will be stacked against you, so having a nice water bottle that will keep your agua cold throughout the shift is a nice way to make hydration a little easier. Some of my colleagues use the motivation bottles and track how much they drink. I'm not that intense (although I may give it a try), so I simply use a 28 oz metal bottle. It is easy to rinse out at the end of the day with the scalding-hot water from the fancy scalding-hot water tap we have at work and I keep it in my locker on some paper towels until the next shift. Note to self: if I've only peed once in a 12-hour shift, perhaps I should drink more water.

Coffee Mug

I will typically drink more coffee in a shift than water. Yes, this is bad. But what would be worse is drinking NO coffee in a shift, as that would have severe repercussions all the way up to the administration of the hospital. A high-quality coffee mug (although I didn't say expensive) can mean the difference between yummy, fresh, sippable happiness and cold, disgusting despair (or a felony). I always find out where I can get good coffee wherever I work and ensure I have the means to keep it hot for those insanely busy shifts.

Snacks

Because you never know when you'll get to eat a meal, you will want to bring some of your favorite snacks with you. I recommend foods that will give you energy and fill you up, as these snacks MAY serve as your breakfast, lunch, dinner, or all three depending on the day. My personal favorites are Clif bars, instant oatmeal, trail mix, peanut butter crackers, and sandwiches (yes, a little ham and cheese or PB&J is a SNACK). I also recommend keeping "emergency" snacks in your bag or locker so even if you run through everything you brought for the day, you have some backup calories should you need them.

Doing Your Homework

Key Research Before You Show Up

Nursing school is long over, but that doesn't mean that you're done taking notes, watching videos, and reading up. Having all the knowledge to be a great nurse isn't the same as knowing what it takes to be a great *employee*. Pay attention during your first few days and make a nice, long list of things you should research to ensure success at your new workplace.

Know the Unit and the Managers

Before arriving on your first day, you should be aware of your unit's purpose within the hospital, the acuity level of the patients there, and the basic structure for management. It is a great idea to enter the job knowing the chain of command. Directing questions to the person who hired you is common as you may be most familiar with him or her, but this person may not be the best resource for your day-to-day questions and concerns. The respectful and responsible thing to do is quickly identify who you will report to and be prepared to use whatever structure the facility has in place to support you. The best way to figure this out is to simply ask.

Finding out about the chain of command is one of my favorite go-to interview questions when applying for a job. "What structure is in place to support me as I begin as a new employee?" "What is the chain of command and who will I report to?" As it is true in most of life, you don't need all the answers–just to know where and how to find them.

Job-Specific Research

Nursing school prepares you for as much as possible, but it is impossible to get expert-level knowledge in specific areas such as trauma, ICU, or ortho in a general nursing program. You must continue your learning and focus on the specialties of your new unit. If you are starting a new job on a neuro unit, for example, you should brush up on your neuro assessments, cranial nerves, and commonly administered medications like TPA and mannitol. A great resource here is your preceptor. Ask what topics you should study up on based on what is most commonly treated on your unit.

New nurses should always carry notecards or a small notebook to write down conditions, tests, and procedures they need to research. When I began working in cardiology, I had a page filled with procedures like AV node ablations, TAVRs, and cardiac caths by the end of my first week at work. I was then able to research these procedures, watch videos on Youtube, and read the hospital care notes about them so I was better prepared to teach and take care of my patients. One of the best educational resources I've found is the collection of patient discharge packets. Our hospital uses a Carenotes database which provides easy-to-read packets on nearly every medication, procedure, and medical condition so we can print them for our patients. I now refer to those discharge packets myself any time I need quick reference information.

Find out what lab values are most important to the work you will be doing on your unit and memorize them. While working with heart failure patients, it is important to monitor kidney function and electrolyte balance because we often treat them with powerful diuretics. I quickly learned what the heart failure team (not my NCLEX review guide) considered normal ranges for potassium and magnesium and at what point we would hold diuretics for elevated creatinine and BUN. I kept these values scribbled down in my notecards until I had them committed to memory. Badge buddies with lab value cheat sheets are another good idea if you don't mind spending a few extra dollars for them.

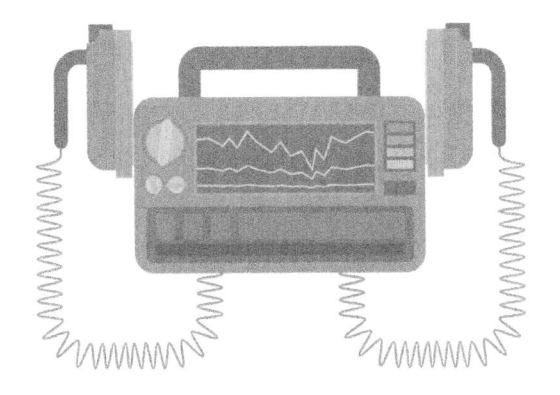

Your First Hours on the Job

Finding Your Way Around

First things first: find the best bathrooms. Your shifts are long and cafeteria food is sometimes questionable. That said, you should make finding both the nearest AND the nicest/most private bathrooms a priority. I'm not going to lie...sometimes I feel like a secret agent sneaking down to the on-call bathrooms when I need a little extra porcelain time.

      You should also find out where and when to get food/coffee. You can't work without fuel in your system, so knowing where to find some calories and/or caffeine is just as important as knowing where the satellite pharmacy is. Your options may depend on your shift times, so make sure you know the hours that certain areas are available to you and plan your day accordingly. Never hesitate to jump on board with coworkers if they are getting take-out, even if you've brought your lunch from home. It is a good opportunity to sample local hotspots that the staff already rely on.

      As I mentioned earlier, make sure you always have some snacks and water with you in case food is inaccessible or you don't have the time to leave your unit to buy something to eat. It's always better to pack more food than you think you'll need. There will be shifts when you're either too busy, you have a patient you cannot walk away from due to his or her acuity, or there simply isn't enough staff to cover you while you leave to grab a meal. In these instances, a few granola bars can save your day, so load up your snack bag.

DIY Phone Directory

Throughout your shift, you will need to call various departments, specialists, doctors, and other units. It will take time to memorize all the phone numbers and extensions that you'll be using, so having a quick reference handy is a gigantic time-saver. I typed up an extension list on a small piece of paper that I taped to my badge buddy for quick reference. When you're brand new, you won't be keen on which numbers you'll use most often but it's a good idea to include any number you could need in an emergency. For me, this included the emergency department, CT scan, the on-call fellows, pharmacy, and security.

You should also always know how to call a code. With 100% certainty. At all times. So write it down and have it accessible.

Michelle Lasota, RN says "Take notes for yourself- start with learning your co-workers' names. That may sound funny but can be overwhelming in the beginning. It is much more difficult to ask for help with anything if you don't know anyone's name. That includes all staff - ex: IT, maintenance, cafeteria staff,

> the lab, etc. Treat everyone with the same respect! We all need each other! Write codes down to the bathroom, linen, clean & dirty utility closets, supply room, and the phone number to your floor- silk tape is your friend! Put a piece on the back of your ID and write all the codes on it - trust me- you're welcome."

ALWAYS know where the crash cart is

From the moment you clock in on your first day, you are an RN at that hospital and certain things are expected of you. This includes the ability to assist in the event of an emergency, even if it is simply helping with patient-moving, CPR, or obtaining supplies. Knowing the location of your unit's crash cart trumps all of the other information you'll absorb on your first day. It is also a good idea to know where oxygen and airway supplies are located as well as the process for obtaining emergency medications.

> Marissa Dovell, RN says "You need to know where all the important stuff is on the unit, including the crash cart and emergency medications. If you're asked to get something in an emergency, you'd

better know where to look. If you don't know, speak up rather than wasting precious time blindly searching the entire unit."

Find the pharmacy, supply department, and CT department

In the same spirit of always knowing where the crash cart is located, I strongly recommend knowing where the pharmacy, supply department, blood bank, and CT scanner are in your facility. In an emergency, you may need to get to one or more of these areas quickly. Knowing in advance the quickest route to get there is a smart move and can be learned easily by taking a few minutes each shift to walk from your unit to each location until you're confident you won't get turned around. If there is any free time during your day, ask your preceptor to send you on a scavenger hunt for these and other important locations around the hospital. Aside from being able to navigate around the hospital, these trips can also put you in front of the hospital staff and give you the chance to begin learning who works where. Don't ever miss an opportunity to introduce yourself and make connections.

Write Down Names

Your first few shifts are going to be a whirlwind of new faces. Rather than being overwhelmed trying to remember everyone, grab your notepad and start writing down names. As you meet doctors, pharmacists, phlebotomists, and therapists write their names down in your notes so you can reference them later. Building rapport with your new colleagues is important and you may end up impressing someone if you can recall his or her name without the awkward glance down at their ID badge. Use names as often as you can and you will prompt your coworkers to pay more attention to you, remember you, and when the time comes, support you as you care for your patients.

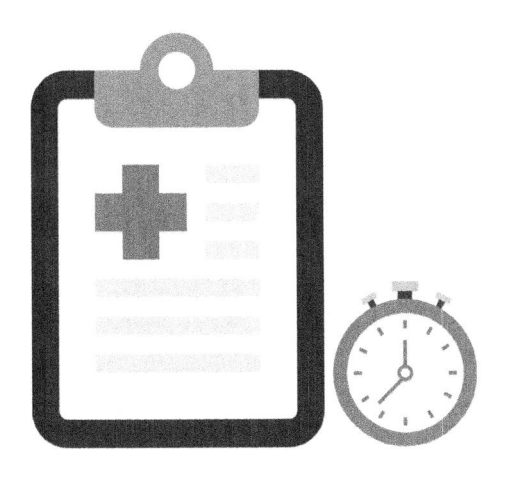

Get Yourself Organized

Begin Establishing a Routine

It took several years to develop and hone my system of organization. I struggled with getting my work done when there were so many chatty patients and coworkers (and I'm no slouch when it comes to chitchat). Prioritizing was difficult and I sometimes forgot important steps when providing care. For instance, I sent a patient to the OR and he still had his boxers on under his gown, which was a no-no. The OR charge nurse made me walk across the hospital, get buzzed into the OR, pick up the patient's underwear which they had kindly removed and bagged for me, and walk them back to my unit. I now refer to this as the Walk of Shame. Was it as bad as when I failed to remove my 70-year-old female patient's nipple rings before her cardiac cath? Arguably.

Eventually, I became much more focused, started to move with urgency, and I developed systems (my fancy way of saying I use a lot of sticky notes) so I wouldn't forget important details. Everyone needs their own personal system of organization but, when you are brand new, it helps to learn from other nurses on the unit in the same way you might use a template. I always tell my orientees that, for the first few days, they should do exactly as I do in terms of organization and routine. This frees up their minds for all the other tasks and concepts they'll encounter and offers them a "trial period" with my system. If they like it, they can keep it…don't like it, toss it for a different system. You will end up creating your own method of doing things by taking pieces from everyone you work with. Use the best, toss the worst, and when you must, create your own.

Ray Lawton, RN says "Take notice of everybody's routine. Note the differences and the similarities and use that to come up with your own from that day forward."

Sticky Notes

Whether you're like me and you use sticky notes or you prefer a notepad, clipboard, or even apps on your computer desktop, keeping a to-do list through your shift is a great way to stay organized, visually plan out your workflow, and prevent forgetting important tasks. I begin my day with Sticky Note #1 which I make at the start of the shift while reviewing my patients. This note contains all of the medications and supplies I'll need to make my morning rounds and saves me from countless trips to the med or utility room. Sticky Note #2 is made during my rounds and contains any requests from my patients, tasks I give myself such as prepping a patient for an upcoming procedure, or reminders to follow up with doctors or specialists based on my morning assessments. Throughout the day, I create a new sticky note anytime a task comes up so I can ensure it will get done regardless of what distractions may pull my attention away.

Timers

That incredibly powerful smartphone in your pocket, and possibly the even more extraordinary little smartwatch on your wrist, have an often overlooked tool to help you stay organized: an alarm clock. I use my phone or Apple watch timer and alarm clock so much throughout the day, it's a wonder that nurses ever got by without them. Timed medications? Prep a patient by 12:45 for a 13:00 procedure? Next PTT to be drawn 6 hours after the last one resulted? No problem, I'll have my assistant take care of it. Hey Siri?

Make Cheat Sheets

I mentioned at the beginning of the book that my wife Marissa is also a nurse. What I didn't mention is just how good she is. Marissa is a hell of a nurse and a master of organization and time management. When she was in her orientation period, she created a one-page "cheat sheet" reference guide for working on her unit. This guide included steps for medication loads, important lab values, ECG measurement thresholds, and what doctors to call for specific issues. Another nurse saw her guide and asked for a copy, and now several years later, it's an unofficial addition to everyone's orientation paperwork on that unit.

You won't know exactly what to put on your cheat sheet on your first day, but you absolutely will be taking notes all day long. Keep these notes organized and, after a few weeks or months, you'll be able to put together your own cheat sheet to keep handy. Some things I added to my cheat sheet are little checklists for transferring patients to other hospitals, sending open-heart patients to the OR, and setting up for a blood transfusion. I also include protocols so I can be a good little nurse and follow my hospital's guidelines for events like hypoglycemia, code sepsis, or an activated fire alarm. They proved helpful even after I had more experience under my belt because, just like my sticky notes, it was a failsafe to keep me from forgetting something important because of distraction.

Find Your Rhythm

Managing time is one of the most challenging elements of your orientation. I recall ending my shift exhausted and frustrated that I ran out of time and couldn't do all of the things I set out to do for my patients. After this happened a few times, I asked Marissa, the Master of Nursing Efficiency, what I was doing wrong. Once I walked her through my day and my process, she identified a few areas where I could greatly improve and, the next shift, I worked on those areas. My rhythm is now much more efficient and I am usually able to balance my workflow as a result.

> *Bill Case, RN, says: "Prepare your cart before the med run and spend less time looking for meds during the run."*

When I am precepting new nurses, I preach that they must come out of the gate strong. This means we get through report and immediately get to work with urgency. Sticky Note #1 is made and we gather everything we will need for the morning in one single trip. We sort meds and double-check we have everything by looking at the patients' charts on our computer, then we start hitting one room at a time.

The first interaction in the morning with each patient is caring, but it is also prompt and direct. I teach my cadence, which I have perfected: "Good morning Mr. Smith, my name is Dave and I'll be the nurse taking care of you today. I have your morning medications and will be giving you a quick check-up. May I see your wristband, please?" That is the script. If my patient is not in distress, it doesn't change. I scan, and I'm back at my medcart scanning meds. There is no casual chatter, I don't ask how the hashbrowns are (they're never good anyway), and I get through the med pass *efficiently*. After a thorough assessment and flushing the IV, I'm back in the hallway again jotting down notes on Sticky Note #2.

    I love being a nurse and caring for my patients, but on my unit with six patients, there is simply no time for pillow-fluffing or coffee refills. We have nursing assistants that will typically round after morning vital signs to provide AM care and turn-downs for our patients anyway, so any comfort request during MY morning rounds gets the same response, "No worries, our nursing assistants are making their way around and can take care of that for you." It's not bad customer service; it's good time management. After all, lives are at stake. Every patient on my team is a life I'm responsible for, so completing my rounds takes priority over providing warm blankets and graham crackers.

So why am I rushing through my morning? Well, rushing implies I may be careless and that is far from the truth. Haste makes waste, not to mention mistakes or missed assessments can be harmful to patients, so I do not *rush*. I am efficient and I avoid wasting time, even a second or two, at all costs as I complete my morning rounds. See, even if everything goes perfectly right, which it most certainly will not, I will barely have enough time in the day to get my work done. By starting strong and completing these morning rounds by, say, 0900, I can free up the remainder of my morning for documenting, sipping coffee, and tackling the work I've laid out for myself on Sticky Note #2.

> *Bill Case, RN, says: "My tennis coach taught me to get to the ball fast and take time with the stroke. Give yourself time to master procedures. With the exception of codes, you have time to do it right. Never feel you have to rush; your timing will improve!"*

Efficiency in the morning also means you will have time later in the day to be present for your patients who need you the most. This is where my guilt came from during my first few shifts: I was too busy to peek in on my elderly "Nervous Nelly" scheduled for a valve replacement in a few days. I was too busy to help explain her procedure in greater detail and to reassure her. I got distracted and forgot to find her a hairbrush so she could feel a bit more human while she waited around with a pit in her stomach. Now, my flow at the start of my shift is efficient. I rifle through tasks smoothly and quickly (not hastily) and avoid wasting time whenever possible. As a result, I create free time in my day to ensure I won't miss a chance to help someone like her again.

> *Tori Meskin, BSN, RNC-NIC says: "Lay a solid foundation of workflow. Try out a few report sheets and find one that works for you. Get the basics down (vital signs, assessments, medications, labs, etc) and build your shift around this. Shifts can get crazy, so starting with a solid foundation to help you manage your shift will help.*

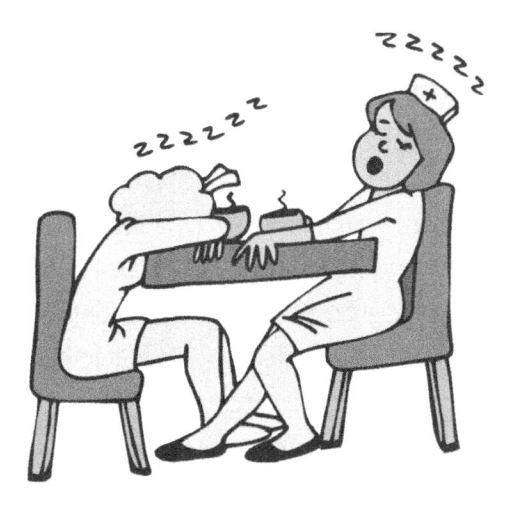

The Night Shift

Special Considerations for Nurse Ninjas

The night shift is a unique working environment for nurses that some love and many can't wait to leave behind for a day shift position. New nurses are frequently started on the night shift as it is less desirable but also tends to be less hectic. While it's true that nurses may enjoy a more laid-back workload on the night shift, it is hardly a fair trade-off for the challenges that come with working while the rest of the world sleeps.

For starters, your family and friends will be up and active while you are drawing the shades to block out the morning sun. Making appointments, running errands, and working with home services like plumbers for a leaky faucet translates to staying up after working all night to get things done. The night shift will mess up your body's circadian rhythm, so you must deliberately find ways to get adequate rest. Working day shift, I typically spread my shifts out throughout the week. When I worked the night shift, however, I would do my best to schedule my 12-hour shifts 3 in a row. This made it easier to get a good sleep in between the shifts while allowing me the time to readjust to night sleeping once my work for the week was done. I spent several years working as a full-time night shifter; here are my tips for conquering the night.

A great way to find balance in your life while working the night shift is by making a weekly time budget. Just like a regular budget, you set portions of time aside for various things like exercise, a hobby, or getting together with family. By sticking to the time budget and holding yourself accountable to the commitments you have made within it, you may find it easier to enjoy the things you love in life while also getting the sleep you need to feel rested at work.

I was quick to discuss my situation with my friends and family once I started working at night. Since I would frequently get invited to functions, holiday dinners, and the like, I reminded my loved ones that my schedule was flipped from theirs. Their noon was my midnight. Even after a few years, it was still common for friends to make cracks about "how late" I would sleep in during my off-days. So they'd get the math lecture, "Look, I got home at 8 am, showered, and was in bed by 8:30. I woke up at 1 pm to get to your house for this barbecue after only sleeping 5 ½ hours! Get off my back."

The first step to prepare for the night shift is when you pack yourself for work. There is less running around at night and many units will drop their thermostats by a few degrees for more comfortable sleeping. You may want to pack a scrub jacket for when things wind down and you get chilly. It's also a good idea to keep a pack-away rain jacket or umbrella in your work bag since you are beginning your shift one day and ending it the next. You never know when you'll end up with a surprise morning rain shower, so best to be prepared.

Aside from your penlight, a small flashlight is useful for checking in on your patients as they rest. I carried two types of lights when I worked on the night shift. One was a USB-powered light that I plugged into the laptop on my WOW. It was just bright enough to illuminate my keyboard and my notes so I could easily work in or around patient rooms without disturbing the patients. The other light was a clip light that I could wear in my scrub top pocket. It had several brightness settings and it was my go-to for peeking in on sleeping patients without waking them.

Food and snacks are harder to come by on the night shift and your hospital may not have a 24-hour cafe. Some hospitals have only vending machines to accommodate the night shift workers. Make sure you load up your nursing bag with plenty of high-energy, high-calorie snacks in addition to packing a nice, big lunch. Caffeine, my personal drug of choice, is great to tote along also, but drink your coffee with consideration of your ability to sleep when the shift is over. I would draw a hard line and cut off all caffeine intake by 2 am to ensure I wasn't tired and wired when I finally got home and crawled under the sheets.

Once you have geared up, it is time to get some quality daytime slumber before your night shift starts. Everyone on the night shift has their own tips and tricks to catch Z's when the sun is shining. Some swear by melatonin supplements while others use white noise machines or play ASMR videos on Youtube. My personal sleep kit includes earplugs, an air purifier that produces just enough white noise to help drown out the daytime din, and high-quality black-out curtains. Sometimes the curtains don't completely block the light, so I pair them with paper black-out shades which can be cut to fit any window and stuck to the window frame with double-sided tape. I also always made sure to put my phone in "do not disturb" mode so my sleep wouldn't be interrupted by kind souls wishing to extend my vehicle's warranty.

More than you ever would when going to bed at night, your bedtime ritual should be set up to truly relax and quiet your mind so you can fall asleep. Make your bedroom a sanctuary that promotes calm and relaxation. Eliminate clutter, use a hamper to hide away laundry, and try to avoid using the room for anything but sleep. An oil diffuser or a lavender candle can add a nice touch of aromatherapy. Splurging on a new mattress and high-quality linens may also improve your ability to fall asleep. If this seems like a lot, just consider how important good sleep is to your physical health and mental well-being. Starting a brand new nursing job is stressful enough without adding the fatigue that comes with sleeplessness. Set yourself up for success before your first night shift even starts and you won't regret it.

When you clock in for your night shift, you may notice the hallways aren't buzzing like they were when you attended your orientation in the daytime. Most of the specialists, doctors, housekeepers, and admins are home for the day, outpatient services are closed, and lights are dimmed. Even in this peaceful environment, your patients are sick. Infections, dysrhythmias, and encephalopathy don't care that it's bedtime so you can't afford to relax. The night shift can be described as 95% laid back and 5% shitshow. Less staff and resources can mean you must be confident in your assessments, think quickly when there are changes to your patient's status, and respond effectively during emergencies.

Most of your patients were probably kept awake all day by consults, tests, scans, and blood draws. By the time the night shift rolls into work, patients have eaten dinner and are ready to get some sleep. Except for the sundowning patient that will require a disproportionate amount of patience and attention, you may spend your shift keeping your patients comfortable and preparing them for whatever tomorrow will bring. I used the night shift to offer more in-depth education to patients requesting it. I would thoroughly review the plan of care for each patient so I could brief the next day shift nurse accurately. The hours after dinner are a great time to ask patients about needs or concerns that you could also bring up in your morning report. Day shift is frequently too busy to get everything done, so I would check to see if patients have documents to sign, DNR orders to renew, special indicator bracelets such as limb alerts were in use, and IVs are not expired. If you can prepare your patients and their charts for the next day, the next nurse will have time to provide higher quality care. Teamwork makes the dream work.

One thing I found to be unique about the night shift is downtime. When I worked the day shift, there was hardly any time to use the restroom in a full 12-hour shift. On the night shift, there were lulls in the activity that allowed me to rest, research patients, and even write some notes for my upcoming blog articles. The problem with downtime is you can become a bit lazy, so I would use checklists to combat this. My "downtime checklist" was a series of tasks to complete which would be much more productive than hiding under a blanket scrolling through Instagram. The list included things like chart checks, restocking med carts, replacing expired IVs, and printing out Carenotes packets to leave on patients' tables. Not only did the checklist make my shift go by much quicker, it kept me focused on my patients so I wouldn't become complacent.

More so than working during the day, the night shift will often allow you to stick much closer to a routine. Once you have established what happens and when on your unit, you may be able to set time goals for your shift. For instance, if I could do my best to finish my med pass and assessments by 2100, documenting would be finished by 22:30 immediately followed by a coffee break. The rest of my routine followed with my checklist, my reassessments, and preparing for the final early morning med pass. There are plenty of times when a late-night admission or an emergency throws off the routine, but usually, it is easy to get back on track once things settle down.

While working the night shift, self-care becomes extremely important to maintain your physical and mental wellbeing. You may not realize it right away, but sleeping through the sunlight, missing chances to be social, and working while most of life is paused takes a toll. Many studies point to night work as carrying an increased risk of diabetes, depression, heart disease, and many other maladies. Don't be afraid to speak up if you feel yourself sliding. Most night-shifters I know, myself included, have gone through periods of lethargy or just feeling down. Isolation and lack of sunlight are used as torture methods for a reason; take time for yourself, make time with friends, family, or your new night-shift colleagues to have fun. Working nights will challenge your ability to balance nearly every aspect of your life, but if you stay in tune with your body and your mental health, you may find that you enjoy the overnight shift.

The night shift may be a perfect starting point for you as a new nurse. The relative consistency of the workflow, ability to follow a routine, and the calmer atmosphere all lend themselves to taking some time to learn the ropes and practice your skills. Do not mistake night shift for being easy, however. Sleeping during the day and working while the rest of the world is dreaming away, paired with the independence of working without hoards of doctors, other nurses, and specialists roaming the hallways makes night shift nursing unique and challenging. It will take a lot of adjustment, planning, and preparation to work at night while staying healthy and productive. Focus as much as you can on getting 8 hours of quality sleep each day, eat right, stay hydrated, and keep your lines of communication open with family and friends.

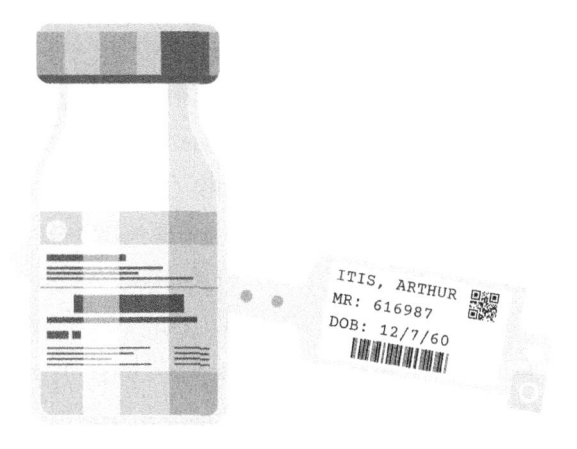

Focus on the Important Stuff

Becoming an Exceptional Nurse

As we discuss the nuances of coffee pots and sticky notes, we can't lose sight of what is most important about nursing. I preach to my brand new nurses that they must practice,

practice, and practice some more with all of their hands-on skills. Muscle memory is so important in nursing and you should make every effort to practice setting up infusions, placing IVs, inserting urinary catheters…practice until every manual skill starts to become second nature. Once you have practiced enough, your hands can do these tasks without much input from your brain. This will free up your mind so it can tackle the higher-level stuff. The important stuff.

> *Cat Golden, RN, says, "Remember that, although you may be new at nursing, you're not new at life! Use skills that help you be successful in your day-to-day life and translate those to your new nursing role. Some examples: maybe you're hilarious and can tell your patients jokes. Maybe you're a great listener or excellent communicator. Whatever your unique skills and abilities are, use those to gain confidence in your new role!"*

Patient Safety

Above all else, it is your responsibility to keep your patients safe. Because we are creatures of habit, I strongly advise you to begin developing good habits concerning patient safety in your first hour on the job. You should ALWAYS identify your patients properly with full names and a secondary identifier. Check every wristband, check the patency of every IV, and make sure the room is safe. An homage to my EMT days, I teach the golden rule: never, ever drop a patient. Do not let your patients fall. Always double-check your medications and drip rates. Be a safe nurse at all times by making safety your number one priority.

When I was an ED tech, I worked with a CT tech who had about 20 years on the job. Everyone in the hospital knew him. A nurse called over to me and said that the patient in Bed 7 was ready for CT so I checked the MAR for an order, checked the patient's wristband, and rolled him down to CT. An hour later, an angry nurse (the same who had asked me to take Bed 7 to CT) tracked me down and asked why I never took her patient. When I explained I did, she rechecked the computer and told me I didn't. I was already in a bit of a mood, so rather than argue I walked over to Bed 7, whipped the curtain open, and said "Sir, remember when I took you to your Cat scan?" He said yes, I asked what the tech looked like, he gave an accurate description. Now the nurse was just simply confused. Where was the scan in the system?

Turns out, the CT tech mixed up which patient had which scan ordered, never checked wristbands and didn't even ask the patient his name. He assumed the patient was someone else and performed the wrong test. What was worse…this mix-up resulted in Bed 7, a renal patient, receiving a heavy dose of IV contrast and prompted the hospital to call in an emergency dialysis team at 3 AM to prevent his kidneys from shutting down completely. The CT tech of 20 years lost his job because he didn't check the patient's wristband. Don't let that be you.

I wasn't sure that I was going to address the recent "escalation" in accountability for nurses that has been headlining the news at the time of this writing. I changed my mind when several colleagues advised me that I couldn't write a book about nursing in 2022 without addressing the elephant in the room. As I sit and type, several nurses sit behind bars after being indicted for varying degrees of negligence that lead to the harm or death of patients. As a strong advocate for both patients and nurses, I am among the many nurses who are torn in their feelings toward this new criminalization of seemingly honest mistakes. As a new nurse, it is rational to read these headlines and wonder just how easy it would be to end up in jail for a mistake of your own.

My reassurance to you will be two-fold. First, remember that of the 4 million nurses in this country, the instances of nurses facing a criminal investigation when there is no criminal intent are extremely rare. Second, you have the advantage of knowing criminal charges are a potential consequence of gross negligence. This knowledge is something the nurses who are presently being charged or sentenced did not have as this is a brand new concept.

As with any tragedy, we must not ignore the positives that come out of this seemingly dark hour for nursing. Always keep the importance of patient safety on the top of your mind for every shift. When in doubt, safety first. This goes for all those little judgment calls you will make throughout the day. "Should I monitor the patient during transport?" If you have to ask, then yes. "Should I place my patient on swallow precautions because he coughs when he takes his pills?" Safety first. If you don't know, ask the doctor and *document*. Take your time, follow protocols, and communicate with your colleagues at every turn. Be sure to take extra time to document your actions so there will be no doubt that you provide safe, quality care to each of your patients. People are relying on you to keep them and their loved ones safe. Do not take this responsibility lightly.

Assessment

Nurses become experts in patient assessment, but this does not happen overnight. It will take time, experience, and the development of a sixth sense to become truly exceptional with assessment. Because you are new and haven't had the time to hone this sense, your assessments should be as thorough as possible. Pay attention to patients and learn the big difference between "sick" and "not sick." Learn to watch out for acute changes in both the physical and mental condition of your patients and never hesitate to call for help or a second set of eyes if you are unsure about something. Eventually, your intuition (and the hairs on the back of your neck) will tell you if something is wrong but in the meantime perform as many head-to-toe assessments as you can. If you have a sick patient who you are genuinely concerned about, position yourself close to that patient at all times. Rather than charting in the back nursing station, I'll slide a computer right up to the patient's doorway and document. Don't trust that his or her condition won't change quickly when you turn your back.

Honesty

Nurses are respected professionals and members of the community. To do our jobs, we must be trusted by our patients, their loved ones, the doctors and specialists, and our colleagues. This trust is built predominantly on the honesty and integrity of nurses all over the world. Help yourself and the profession of nursing by being honest at all times. Don't make promises you can't keep. Don't let your pride get in the way of admitting when you don't know something. Don't be a storyteller and don't use your imagination when explaining things to your patients, doctors, or other providers.

Most importantly, acknowledge your mistakes and report them immediately. Even though nurses appear to be superhuman, we are capable of making mistakes like anyone else. As scary as it sounds, you WILL slip up at some point or another. Most hospitals have now adopted a non-punitive environment for reporting errors to improve patient safety and outcomes. If you give the wrong medication or dose, send the wrong patient for a test, or make any other mistake, take a deep breath and own it. Reporting a mistake immediately could potentially prevent harm to your patient, so there should be no hesitation about coming forward quickly and working toward a resolution.

Integrity

One of my nursing school instructors described integrity as being the way you act when no one is watching. As nurses, we are trusted to work safely, properly, and cleanly even when no one is around. If you are willing to cut corners and do whatever you could get away with, you undoubtedly should find a new career. Regardless of whether you are in front of coworkers, patients, and family members or working alone behind a closed door, the way you conduct yourself should be the same. Drop a pill on that filthy hospital floor and no one saw? Waste it and get a new one. IV bag with the patient's name on it is empty and the shredder bin is on the other side of the unit? Rip that label off and walk it to the bin. Your altered patient soiled himself for the third time in your shift? Speak with caring and compassion regardless of whether he can understand you. Always assume your patients can hear you no matter their condition. Don't build a habit of taking shortcuts or working dirty– that is NOT putting your patients first. Moral character is everything and your patients are counting on you to always do right by them; don't let them down.

Advocacy

When my patients express distrust toward their doctors, other nurses, or are uncomfortable with anything pertaining to their care, I always remind them that I work for my patients first. My nursing license says "Registered Nurse," not "This Hospital's Employee" or "Dr. Jones' Personal Assistant." I always put my patients and their needs above all else and will go to bat for them wherever necessary. Show your patients respect and stick up for them. It is never your place to judge them even when they may be unpleasant to care for. Go the extra mile whenever you can and remember that, while this may simply be another shift for you, you could be caring for this patient during the worst time of his or her life.

One communication tool to use when advocating for your patients is called CUS words. No, I'm not referring to the blatant yet creative profanity I use which causes my coworkers to shut the door to the nursing lounge whenever I open my mouth. I'm talking about CUS the acronym which stands for Concerned, Uncomfortable, and Safety. CUS is a way to escalate your concerns for your patient in a professional way.

An example of using CUS would be if your patient has a blood pressure that continues to trend higher each day since admission but the treatment team is not intervening. You call the doctor and explain the situation, "The patient's blood pressure was 150/88 on arrival and has since trended up to 180/92. There have been no changes to the patient's medications and I am CONCERNED." If the physician blows it off and remarks that they will look into the issue during rounds tomorrow morning, you can escalate and say, "I am UNCOMFORTABLE that the patient's blood pressure continues to rise without any interventions. Is there something I can do for him now?"

Hopefully, by this point, the doctors will evaluate the patient and place orders, but in the event they do not, you can escalate further. "This is a SAFETY issue for my patient." Once an issue reaches this point, you will typically have to bring in your charge nurse, nursing supervisor, and other team members into the loop to reach a resolution for the patient. Don't be afraid to do this! You are doing your job and keeping your patients safe which is way more important than trying to avoid confrontation. Patient advocacy is right in our job description and your patients are relying on you to be their voice.

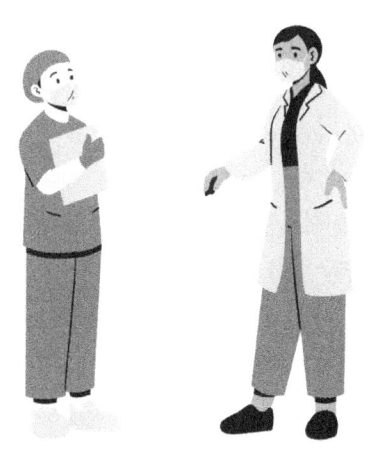

Meet Your Preceptor

Buddying Up with Your Numero Uno

Few people will be as influential as your preceptor during your first few months as a nurse. Most new nurses will orient for 8-12 weeks or so and, during this time, their preceptor will show them the ropes and help them adjust to the facility. It is important to establish a good rapport with your preceptor right off the bat. Every preceptor will have a different style and different philosophy when it comes to your orientation. Some may be very hands-on and treat you like a baby brother or sister while others may have more of a trial-by-fire approach. You may not click right away with your preceptor or her style, and that's okay! I suggest giving a bit of time before getting discouraged; you both may adapt to each other and have a great experience. Either way, it is important to always remain professional and communicate with your preceptor to ensure you have an optimal and educational orientation period.

> *Michelle Clarke, RN says "I know an orientee is good when I see that they are asking questions and taking notes, actively seeking learning opportunities, and show a willingness to help both patients and coworkers."*

A preceptor's job is to acclimate you to the facility and the unit, help you manage your workflow, and serve as a resource when you have questions. He or she will not expect you to have all the knowledge you need on your first day, but this doesn't mean you aren't responsible for competency. From your first day, your patients are your responsibility and you are providing care for them using the license you worked your butt off to get. Leaning on your preceptor is okay when necessary, but don't expect him or her to pick up your slack.

> *Bill Case, RN, says: "I think it's tempting not to ask questions. You don't want to bother people or be a pest. Or you don't want to look needy. Some people encourage questions while others want you to figure things out the way they did when no one helped them. Asking questions makes you an active learner, benefits everyone, and confirms/reinforces your understanding of the task."*

A good preceptor will be comfortable communicating with you to find out your strengths and weaknesses, as well as having the ability to pick up on your learning style. If you believe your preceptor is on a different wavelength than you, it is best to address this openly, professionally, and always with the clear objective of getting better each day as a new nurse.

Being a "Good" Orientee Tips

- DON'T think or act like you know everything.
- DON'T guess that you are doing something properly. If you are unsure, ask your preceptor if you can walk through a process with them and they can correct any missteps.
- DON'T be an unsafe nurse.
- DON'T participate in workplace gossip or group complaining.
- DO listen more than you speak.
- DO fill every moment of downtime by learning or helping on the unit.
- DO take the initiative.
- DO express any concerns immediately with your preceptor before they become larger problems.
- DO keep a positive attitude. If you're having a rough day, the time to vent is <u>after</u> your shift.

As you meet and get to know your preceptor, keep an open mind and a positive outlook. The fact alone that she took the courses and training to become a preceptor in the first place is an indication that she enjoys helping new nurses become successful. It may not always seem like it, but your preceptor is on your team.

There are cases where the relationship between a preceptor and orientee becomes so abrasive that it simply doesn't work out, but this is very rare. Your preceptor will typically go above and beyond for you to help in any way she can. If you're unsure after a few days if your preceptor is a "good fit" for you, avoid jumping to negative conclusions. Working with a variety of personalities is a part of being a professional nurse, so maintain a positive mindset.

> *Michelle Clarke, RN says "I do not expect a new nurse to know everything, but I do expect them to know what they don't know and ask questions. I fully expect that a new nurse will be a bit slow in the beginning, and that's okay. I would much rather they be overly cautious to start."*

I recall filling in to precept an orientee when her assigned preceptor had to call in sick for the shift. Since I was unfamiliar with just how much the orientee was capable of on her own, I stayed with her throughout the morning and was never farther than arm's reach if she needed help. By lunchtime, she expressed to me that her preceptor let her go off on her own most of the day and was often difficult to find when she had questions or needed help. Rather than continue working in a way that was making her orientation experience difficult, my advice to the orientee was to open the line of communication with her preceptor and explain exactly what her comfort level is. Later that week, they had a conversation and the orientee simply explained she would prefer if her preceptor could stay in the hallway outside her patients' rooms and be accessible should she have questions. Her preceptor agreed and the problem was solved without issue.

> *Wanda Goodmond, RN says*
> *"Understand that, because you just graduated, you have fresh knowledge that the seasoned nurse may not have, so share it! You AND your preceptor will learn something new every day.*

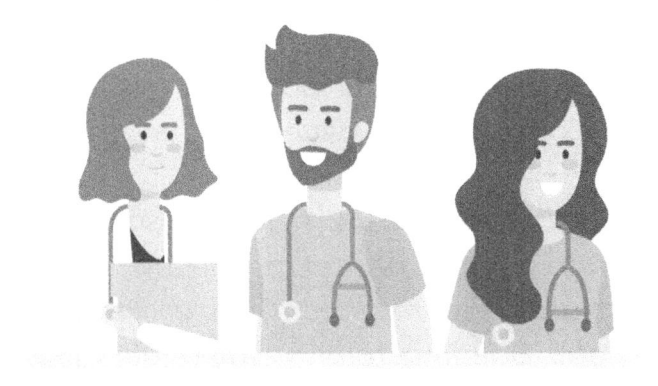

Building Relationships

Getting to Know Your Future Work Family

Well, here they are: the men and women that you will work, laugh, cry, and spend holidays with. Being the "new nurse" can be intimidating just like entering into any new social situation. Face it, everyone in that building knows one another better than they know you. Yet, this is such an exciting opportunity to make connections, establish yourself as a professional, and garter positive relationships to benefit both your work life and the outcomes of your patients.

> *Tori Meskin, BSN, RNC-NIC says: "Get to know your unit. I'm talking everyone. Nurses, secretaries, CNA or Techs, MDs, etc. Building relationships will help you navigate your shift, increase confidence from your team members, and ultimately help you in your patient care."*

Yes, your interactions with other members of the staff will have a direct impact on how well you can care for patients. Nursing is a team sport and, without teammates, you just aren't playing it right. So be friendly, positive, and build good relationships early on with your new coworkers so they will be there for you and your patients when push comes to shove. It is truly the teamwork that will make or break your day working as a nurse.

Nursing Assistants and Techs

Each role in the hospital contributes to the care of patients and it is often the nurse who must coordinate all of the other specialists.

Developing a healthy rapport with nursing assistants and patient care techs should be one of your primary focuses when you begin your first nursing job. Your hardworking CNA can be a wealth of knowledge, knows all the tips and tricks, and can drag your shiny new self through the most challenging shifts.

If you expect to be well-received by your new teammates, treating ancillary staff with respect and professionalism is mandatory. Pay attention to how hard they work and acknowledge it often. Show gratitude and include them in everything from ordering out for lunch to making outside-of-work plans. If you are there for the nursing assistants, techs, and others who support you, they'll be there for you when you need them most.

> *Gabrielle Corbin, PCT says "Nurses and techs should understand that we are all here to help each other. We need to communicate with each other to make things run smoothly."*

While delegation is a part of your job, do so conscientiously. A big no-no is to pawn off an unpleasant task to your nursing assistant or patient care tech while you sit back and enjoy a coffee break. Never ask for help, then sit on your ass! That aid or tech will feel used and abused and you can quickly lose his or her respect. Much worse, word will spread quickly among the other aids and techs. Before you know it, you'll be cruising past so many cold shoulders on your unit that you'll need a sweater.

Communication with your aids and techs should be effective and not demanding. Early on, I found that I had not yet proven myself as a hard worker to the support staff. I went out of my way a bit when I communicated to clarify tasks I wanted to delegate during this time. For example, rather than "Could you help Mr. Jones onto a bedpan?" I would ask, "Emily, I'm a bit behind on my meds. Could you please help Mr. Jones onto a bedpan while I get caught up?" This communication would be followed up later with, "Thank you so much, Emily. I was able to get all caught up while you helped Mr. Jones." I would go out of my way to explain *why* I was delegating a task and, in a way, was telling my aid or tech "Hey, trust me, if I could get this done myself, I would. But I can't, so let's divide and conquer." If this seems silly or simple to you, that's okay. But I challenge you that if you start working and you notice your aids and techs are less-than-enthusiastic to help you when you ask, revisit this section and see if you are communicating effectively and with appreciation.

> *Gabrielle Corbin, PCT says "New nurses sometimes believe certain things are 'below their pay grade' and will waste more time to track us down than to simply do the task themselves. Teamwork is a two-way street. Out of respect, if you see your tech is running around but nurses aren't busy, ask if you can do anything to help out."*

Befriending the Unit Coordinator

The secretary or unit coordinator often fields your phone calls, can reach out to docs and other disciplines for you, and helps organize the flow of patients for you. Treat this hero like gold. A decent unit coordinator will have his or her finger on the pulse of the unit at all times and usually gets plenty of facetime with unit managers, nursing supervisors, and other decision-makers. You owe it to your patients to build a healthy relationship with the coordinator because oftentimes she can make a big difference in the flow of your day.

Where I work, the unit coordinators answer calls from procedure areas, imaging, and the ORs regarding our patients. They play the role of the middle person, often tracking us down and relaying information on our behalf. This is a huge time-saver for our nurses but not necessarily a job requirement for the coordinator. It's not something she *has* to do for you, and neither is shouting out phone extensions for the doc you need or sending your fax to another department. In other words, she can make your shift a living hell if she wanted to. So, if you're a big DIY person, go ahead and get on your unit coordinator's bad side; I guarantee you'll be doing much more yourself.

Doctors

Every hospital has a different culture, so you'll have to get a feel for the doctor-nurse relationship where you work. I have worked in facilities where physicians avoid eye contact with anyone who isn't another doctor. I have also worked in places where the doctors learn your name, joke around with you, and have your back when you need it. Hopefully, your new job will be like this, but some universal tips will help you establish rapport with the medical staff either way.

Be prepared to answer questions. When discussing a patient with doctors, learn to anticipate their questions and have answers ready to go. For instance, don't go calling a doctor about your patient's chest pain without already assessing, obtaining vitals, and checking to see what medications the patient is taking or has available. In most facilities, the protocol would allow you to also obtain an ECG and possibly give medications such as nitroglycerin or aspirin.

What a doctor wants to hear is a modified or shortened SBAR (Situation, Background, Assessment, Recommendation) like the one in the example below:

> "It's Dave from the Cardiology Unit. Do you know Mr. Smith in Room 3? No? Okay, so Mr. Smith in Room 3 was admitted yesterday for worsening shortness of breath and is waiting for a heart failure consult. He has new-onset substernal non-radiating chest pain he describes as sharp and burning. He is normal sinus on the monitor, vital signs are within normal limits, we put him on 2

liters of oxygen and gave 1 nitro with no relief. The patient does have a history of GERD but is not currently on any PPIs. Would you like an EKG?"

This report briefed the doctor, regardless of whether he is familiar with the patient or not, on why the patient is here and what is going on that requires his or her attention. You painted a picture quickly and, using your nursing intuition, guided the doctor by mentioning pertinent information. Reflux could present as cardiac pain, so bringing up the patient's history of GERD and suggesting it as a differential makes sense. You are also indicating that you have already started your hospital's protocol for acute chest pain and that you'd like to obtain an EKG to move the process along. This 30-second "SBAR" report provides enough of the big picture to the doc without being convoluted by unnecessary information.

As doctors get to know you, they will take your advice, suggestions, and requests seriously. This is great for your patients because you will get to know what they truly need and, if your reputation with the doctors is solid, you'll be able to get whatever you need for your patients quickly. To start building this trust with the docs, make *educated* requests when discussing a patient.

I had an NPO patient who was complaining about how thirsty she was. Armed with my vast knowledge from nursing school and fueled by a drive to advocate for my patient, I immediately called the doctor and asked for IV fluids to rehydrate her. The doc sighed and reminded me the patient had heart failure, volume-overload, and was getting IV Lasix twice a day. I felt like an ass.

You should always punctuate your calls to the doctors with a request, but make sure you think it through. Don't ask for a medication the patient is allergic to, don't ask for contraindicated scans, and if you REALLY don't know what to ask for, my favorite line is: "I really don't feel comfortable with the patient's status, could you come to see the patient?" The doctors went to school for a long time and accumulated a significant amount of student debt so they could know what to do for their patients; get them brainstorming with you!

Don't apologize! So many nurses begin their call to a doctor by saying, "Hi Dr. Jones, it's Dave. Sorry to bother you…" Or "I'm sorry, but…" If there is one piece of advice I was given as a new nurse that stuck with me, it would be when Wanda Goodmond, RN told me that <u>I wasn't sorry.</u> She explained, "You are helping the doctor by caring for his patient. You are telling him what is going on. You are his eyes and his hands. You are not sorry…you are doing your job."

> *Wanda Goodmond, RN says "Remember: you work with the doctor, not for the doctor. If you are working in a hospital, your paychecks come from the same place. Never apologize for a phone call, a question, or an observation. Try not to be intimidated, smile, and talk to them. They started just where you're at. You'll be surprised how much you may have in common."*

Management

In most hospitals, management operates a bit further away than you may have experienced in jobs you worked when you were younger. You are a licensed professional and are expected to perform your duties well, keep patients safe, respect your workplace, and govern yourself without micromanagement. But just because you don't interact with your managers every day doesn't mean building a relationship with your leadership team is any less important.

As with all things, a balance is key. Brown-nosing has no place in a professional hospital and can be detrimental to nursing as a profession. Rather, there should be mutual respect between nurses and management as we all wish to provide the best care for patients and enjoy a comfortable life outside of the job. I'll break down my tips for building your relationship with management into a few sections.

Shoot for perfect attendance.

Time off is a critical part of nursing, as it allows you time to rest and recuperate from the struggles that you'll inevitably encounter. This said, as a new nurse, you have the opportunity to establish yourself and build your reputation from the ground up. Frequently calling in sick and booking time off when you are brand new can be detrimental to this reputation. Not only could frequent time off raise a few eyebrows from your management team, but you will also have less continuity in your schedule and may find it more challenging to practice your new job. Try to save your sick days for when you are actually sick. For all of life's other curveballs, see if you can swap shifts with a coworker rather than taking the day off.

Be flexible with your schedule.

Anyone who has ever made a staff schedule will tell you how valuable flexibility is for ensuring all shifts get covered. As a new nurse, your job should rank very high on your priority list, and therefore try to be as flexible as possible with your work schedule. I don't mean you should miss an important life event like a wedding or funeral. Save for a few exceptions, working when you are needed will definitely put you in your manager's good graces.

Meet deadlines for mandatory training.

As a new hire, you will have a huge mountain of training, classes, and computer-based learning to do. I recommend keeping a list of these responsibilities very handy and setting reminders so you do not miss any deadlines. Many of these training activities are put into place by the administration, HR, or the compliance department. If you miss one or are late, these departments will usually see your name in red and with flags in their database.

They'll typically reach out to your unit manager with an email that reads something like this: "Dear Manager, the employee you just hired didn't do the thing she was supposed to do. It's really important that she does, and it's your job to make sure she gets it done. So if you don't want YOUR name on OUR naughty list, make sure she gets it done. Cordially yours, someone in a suit who you may or may not ever actually meet." The moral of the story: stay on your manager's good side and get your classes and training done on time.

Communicate professionally and promptly via email or other approved methods.

Checking your work email can be difficult to remember when you are new and have another million things to worry about. Still, if a manager, educator, or anyone else is trying to communicate with you via email, it can be a bad look to leave them unanswered for 2 weeks because you simply have been neglecting to check for messages. Make a habit of checking your email at a certain time each day (I always like to do it when I return from lunch. If someone else is covering my patients, I can usually check for messages at the same time they are briefing me on anything that happened while I was away.

When writing work emails, be as professional as possible in your writing. Use proper spelling, grammar, and formatting regardless of what you observe from others. Just because your manager may write an email to you as if it is a text message doesn't mean you should do the same. This may be just a personal pet peeve of mine, but I look at emails this way: if all of my emails are professional, I'll never have an issue whereas if they are unprofessional, someone someday may think less of my abilities because I didn't capitalize or included emojis in a work email. Have you heard the expression "dress for the job you want?" That is all about representing yourself the right way; writing emails is the same deal.

Keep in mind this goal as you build your professional relationships: you want your management team to view you as a positive asset to their team. When managers see or hear your name, it should trigger a release of endorphins and they should smile. Again, this doesn't mean you should be a kiss-ass. It means being reliable, responsible, and staying off naughty lists. Why is this so important? One word: opportunities. Nursing is a unique profession with many opportunities that will present themselves throughout your career. Most of these will likely funnel through your leadership team, so keeping yourself on the "good" list will put you at an advantage. These opportunities could come in many forms, such as a chance to become a charge nurse or a preceptor for new nurses. They could also be invitations to work on special committees, fun ways to earn extra money through community outreach and other paid activities, and even winning awards for your hard work. By proving yourself as reliable, flexible, and proficient, you are giving yourself a better chance at these opportunities and more.

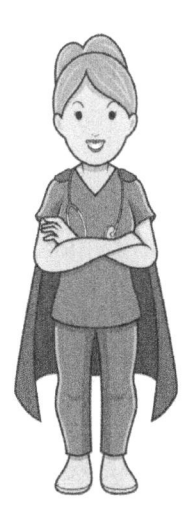

Establishing Your Reputation

First Impressions are Key

As I have mentioned, you are the new nurse. It is your opportunity and responsibility to begin building your reputation. A solid reputation will mean your colleagues trust and respect you, your patients receive what they need to get better, and you will have a lifetime of open doors to step through. Every action you take will either add to or detract from your professional reputation. This doesn't mean you should be afraid to make mistakes or nervous that colleagues won't like you; it means you should always make an effort to put your best foot forward and stay positive.

In the first few minutes on the job, your coworkers will already be sizing you up. This is okay! It's a chance for you to let them know that you are happy to be there, excited to learn, and willing to help. Your appearance and presentation will be very important in helping your workers form a good first impression of you, so be sure your new fancy scrubs are clean and pressed, your hair is neatly done, guys' faces are freshly shaved or neatly trimmed, and for the majority of you who are ladies, do NOT go nuts with your makeup, nails, and smelly stuff. Conservative, clean, and professional is the look you are going for.

Verbal and body language also play a huge role in how your coworkers will perceive you, so be mindful of both. Avoid leaning and sitting at inappropriate times. Good posture ensures people that you are confident. If you walk around all day with your hands in your pockets or your arms folded across your chest, it can be a put-off or make you seem unapproachable. Use positive language, smile when you speak, and (I can't believe I'm saying this) try not to use profanity. Everyone who knows me is shaking their heads, but hear me out. Cursing *when you are new* doesn't set a professional tone. Wait until you are a bit more established to start adding to the swear jar and remember, your patients can hear way more than you think they can. Be constructive with your language, offer genuine compliments, and stay professional. Positivity is contagious and people will subconsciously enjoy working with you if you consistently put out positive vibes.

Nursing is a stressful job and you will be working with a wide range of different personalities. It is unrealistic to think you will get along with every single one of your colleagues. As with everything else, there is a balance to be struck. On one hand, you shouldn't get upset if you don't become best friends with each person you work with. With this in mind, you do have to consider your patients, your career, and your professional image before getting into any sort of altercations or arguments with your coworkers. My advice is to always play nice, keep a positive attitude, and be the bigger person in all circumstances. Despite being brand new, it won't be long before YOU are the nurse all of the new grads are looking up to. It's never too early to practice being a role model.

> *Michelle Lasota, RN says "Most importantly, learn the difference between reacting and responding! Many things will trigger your emotions and leave you wanting to react - instead, take a few very deep breaths, even walk away for a few minutes if needed, process your emotions and think of how you would like to respond! This will yield a big difference in the outcome of your scenario."*

The best reputation to have on your unit is that of a team player, so do your best to help out when you have time. Nursing shifts are long and tiring, even when everything goes right. The rare moment to take a break is something you'll want to savor, but it can be hard to sip coffee when your colleagues are "in the weeds". This is where being an efficient nurse comes in. Your efficiency will afford you both the opportunity to help your coworkers AND take small breaks if you plan things right. Avoiding chitchat, clustering care, and remaining focused through your daily duties are all great ways to save time. It's a wonderful feeling to know that you have enough time in your day to take exceptional care of your patients, help your fellow nurses a bit, AND enjoy a bit of downtime on the shift to use the bathroom or get something to eat.

Remember: what goes around typically comes around. If you are the nurse that is ALWAYS too busy to help your coworkers in a pinch, they will be less likely to jump and save your backside when you need it most. While you will probably be so busy in your first few shifts you'll barely keep your head above water, you should still avail yourself to be a team player whenever possible.

> *Michelle Lasota, RN on hard work: "I firmly believe in maintaining a strong work ethic - however, you must know that not everyone will model the same ethic or place the same value on their work as you. Never decrease your work ethic to match something less than you believe your standard of care to be. Rather, continue moving forward and set the example for the change you want to see. This is not always an easy*

thing to do BUT you need to walk away from each day feeling like you did the best you could with the challenges you faced."

Another way to assimilate into the culture at your new job is to offer yourself. You will have tons of opportunities working as a nurse to step out of the normal routine of patient care. Part of becoming a team player in your new workplace is participating in other activities when they arise. Most hospitals have a variety of committees to join and some even require membership in at least one or two.

Ways to get involved:

- Join committees
- Start a committee if you see a need
- Write for the newsletter
- If your hospital performs research, find out how you could get on a project team
- Become a "superuser" for a piece of equipment or software
- Sign up for community outreach
- Take continuing education classes if they are offered
- Find out if you could become a CEU course instructor
- Become a BLS/ALS instructor
- Sign up for community outreach

Important to note: while there may be a hundred different ways to engage with your workplace and your colleagues, it can be easy to say "yes" too easily and get stretched too thin. Don't get taken advantage of because everyone assumes they can toss something your way and it will get done. Before taking on a new activity or role, carefully consider what impact the time commitment will have on your job, other activities, and time away from work. Balance is key and if you find you are becoming overwhelmed, it is time to cut your workload.

Equally important, it is possible to be "too helpful" while at work. Whether that is in the form of running around the unit like a tornado trying to do too much or by simply always saying yes to helping out and neglecting your own patients (or even yourself). On one side of a very fine line is being helpful and ambitious. On the other side is being over-worked or taken advantage of. Are you this person? Ask yourself some basic questions to find out.

- How many times have I gone to the bathroom today?
- Did I have lunch?
- Will I stay at work an extra 2 hours today to finish my charting?
- Am I drinking enough water?

If you are troubled by your answers to any of these questions, it might be time to reevaluate your workflow and ask your coworkers to reciprocate all the favors you've been providing. Being too much of a people-pleaser can be exhausting and detrimental to the people who matter the most: *your patients.*

> *Michelle Lasota, RN says "Always offer to lend a hand to a fellow coworker when someone needs help turning, bathing, repositioning a patient, or assistance with wound care, running to grab supplies...don't hesitate to offer the help. This shows you are willing to be a team player, to learn whenever the opportunities present themselves, and to take initiative. Most importantly, when you are suddenly the person who needs an extra hand, you will have established comradery with your co-workers who will want to return the favor. Remember! People may not remember your name right away, but they will never forget how you made them feel."*

Cell Phone Culture

Shifting to another simple way to ensure you don't develop a bad reputation right off the bat is to stay off your phone. We are living in the 21st century and colleagues of all ages and experience levels are aware of just how powerful our smartphones are. It would be unrealistic and irresponsible to think we would be toting around such a resource in our pockets without ever using it, but *how* we use our phones at work is what could harm our professional reputation.

Don't be tempted by the behavior of your colleagues. If everyone else at the nursing station is watching Tiktoks or messing around with new Snapchat filters, this doesn't mean you should, too. What you don't know is how these colleagues are being perceived by your superiors or peers and what reputation they are establishing for themselves. Your downtime would be much better spent providing extra care to your patients, grabbing a snack for some energy, or getting ahead with your documentation. There is always something to do, so consider making a little "extra checklist" you can consult in your notes for when rare free time presents itself. Do any of your patients need new IVs? Consent forms to be signed? Have you reviewed recent labs and orders? Staying busy with your work results in a better experience for your patients and keeps you out of trouble.

A story from personal experience: While working on my telemetry unit, things calmed down in the late afternoon and I found myself and my fellow nurses huddled around the nursing station on our WOWs documenting and chatting. The nursing supervisor for the shift approached us and checked in, asked how we were all doing, and if we needed anything. We told her everything was going well, we were all caught up…no issues. She puts her clipboard down on the desk and says, "I don't mean to vent, but can I just say how your floor is like night and day to the sixth floor? I was just up there and their call bells were lit up like Christmas trees. The unit was a mess and the nurses were all hiding in the dictation room on their phones while their only nursing assistant was running around like a madwoman." She shook her head, tapped on the desk, and gave us an animated "Thank you," before making her way to the elevator.

By the next shift, the "lazy" nurses from the sixth floor had already earned themselves a new, bad reputation. Fast-forward a few months and one of those nurses applied for an assistant unit manager position. Part of the interview process was a panel interview in front of multiple managers and nursing supervisors who would take turns asking "what would you do if" questions. Of course, one of these supervisors was the one who witnessed the applicant messing around on her phone rather than attending to her patients and, of course, she didn't get the job. The issue came up as the interview panel deliberated and the nurse in question has been blacklisted from any sort of future promotion. As far as we know, she doesn't even know she's been blacklisted or the reason why.

  This is why I preach so much about establishing and maintaining a reputation. Doors will open for you if you are known around the hospital as a helpful, hardworking, reliable nurse. They'll close just as quickly if your colleagues and managers scoff or roll their eyes when your name is mentioned.

Being a Good Orientee

If spending your shift on your phone earns you the label of "lazy nurse," then spouting off every piece of knowledge you acquired from your stack of nursing textbooks will earn you the esteemed title of "know-it-all." Many new nurses are just a few months out of nursing school when they start their first job. With all of this "book knowledge" still fresh in your mind, you may find yourself sharing just how smart you are with your preceptor and other nurses around you as a way to prove your worth. Keep in mind that the nurses around you may not recall every piece of information from your textbooks, especially if they have been out of school for decades. This doesn't mean they aren't experts in their field who can probably find out more about their patients from the doorway than if you studied those patients' charts for 3 hours. Book smarts are no replacement for experience and instincts, so follow their guidance. Try to avoid correcting your fellow nurses, especially in front of others, and don't fall into the false confidence that a 4.0 GPA may have created. Stay humble, keep your mouth closed, and your ears open.

Hospitals are dynamic, emotional workplaces full of all kinds of people and all kinds of issues. Use your first few months to "take it all in" while avoiding criticism, complaining, and staying out of any drama. Some of us will inevitably get ourselves into workplace gossip, so I'll try to remain realistic in the advice I give. Don't get roped into all the gossip and drama when you are new. As enormous as a hospital can be, it has always surprised me just how small of a world it really is. Someone always knows someone else, people are related to one another, dating one another, maybe even married to one another and you don't always know. It is best practice to keep yourself out of the drama and focus on your work, patients, and establishing a professional relationship with your coworkers.

     Complaining about your new workplace (or those in it) is another way you can get yourself into trouble and I advise against it. It can be easy to get caught up in the bitch-fest when your fellow nurses aren't happy about something, but this is another case when keeping that mouth closed is your best option. Shrug and stay busy. The complaining nurses have already built their reputations and their colleagues most likely won't base their opinions of them on a few negative comments. You, on the other hand, have no reputation. If one of the first interactions people have with you is hearing you complain about the manager, other nurses, the facility, or even the patients...they will often form a negative view of you. If you have legitimate concerns about how something is being handled, send them up the chain of command professionally and constructively.

A personal note on "complaining." I am not shy about bringing up concerns at work and suggesting alternative ways to do things. This said, I always focus on the positives and I will come up with a feasible plan to improve the situation. This comes with some experience in management and knowledge of "how the world works." Rather than complaining about how short-staffed the unit is, you might suggest volunteering to lead a retention and recruitment committee. People love problem-solvers, not just someone who points out which problems exist.

Leave your issues at the door.

This can be difficult in nursing, especially if you work 12-hour shifts multiple days in a row. At some point, there will be a time when you have to sneak off the unit for an important phone call or to handle something in your personal life. You will most likely make life-long friends along the path of your career and these people will have your back when times get tough. These relationships will take some time to build, so at the beginning of your career, I would recommend allowing your family life and other influences a minimal impact on your day at work. As best as you can, think of work as a place where you can put any troubles you are having on the back burner and just focus on your patients. With the right mindset, coming to work can actually be a stress reliever and may offer you the time you need to put other issues in your life into proper perspective.

The lump sum of what your new coworkers know about you can be split into two categories: your credentials and your reputation. The credentials speak for themselves and include those two big letters that follow your name, R and N, and all that comes with it. They know you have a nursing degree, passed your boards, and possess a nursing license. They know you are BLS certified and can do CPR if there is an emergency. They know you can perform the skills required by your nursing school program with some degree of competency. Other than that, you are a blank slate. Everything else will rest with the development of your professional reputation, so be conscious and deliberate in how you build yours.

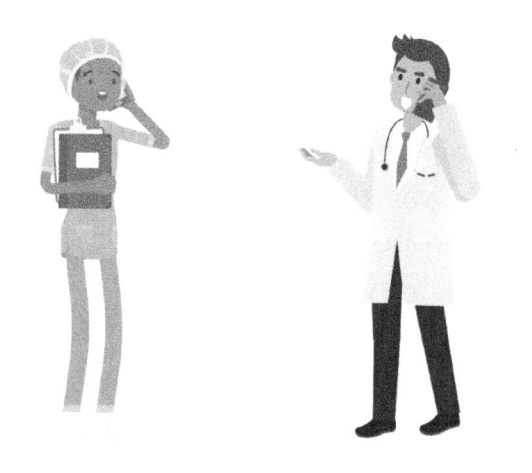

Communicating with your Colleagues

C'mon Now...Use Your Words

Nursing is all about communication. You must be an effective and efficient communicator with your colleagues, charge nurses, managers, unit coordinators, ancillary staff, doctors, and all of the specialists working in your facility. Most will look to you, the nurse, as the first point of contact for a patient. Families will rely on you for updates. Patients will turn to you to explain what is happening and their plan of care in a way they can understand. Keeping notes, remembering to pass along messages, and finding ways to keep everyone on the treatment team up-to-date are all skills you should work on immediately after starting your first job.

      Your colleagues will want to know if you are the type of person they can trust to have their back. This could manifest in many ways, but being someone they can turn to when they need a second opinion, some advice, or someone to vent to can be one of the first ways you connect with your coworkers. Be open and available, keep private information to yourself…just be a good person. Getting to know your coworkers on a personal level will make it easier to deal with the tough, heartbreaking days that we as nurses will inevitably encounter from time to time.

> *Wanda Goodmond, RN says "Honesty and support make a team. Be willing to listen and help. Talk about things that are not work-related; it helps when you know someone and what's important to*

them. Be tolerant because everyone can have a bad day."

Professionally, one of the more stressful lines of communication we use as nurses is between ourselves and the doctors. In nursing school, many of us learned about the SBAR method of communicating with doctors and other providers/specialists. As I mentioned in my section about working with doctors, this method is when you provide the Situation, Background, Assessment, and Recommendation to a doctor when calling about a patient. I can tell you firsthand that the first few times you must call a physician, you may be nervous or think you sound like a dimwit on the phone. You might. But I have some tips that will make your first few phone calls (plus every call after them) go a little easier.

Michelle Clark, RN says "Gather your thoughts first and have your patient information in front of you in case they have questions."

When calling the doc, be sure to keep your conversation short and to the point. Many times, doctors are very busy and your call may have interrupted them. Only provide information *relevant* to the person on the other end of the phone. If you are calling wound care for a consult on a worsening diabetic ulcer, that person probably doesn't need to know what day the patient had a coronary stent placed, which vessel it was, and what type of stent was used. If it helps, plan your call on a sticky note and jot down some *relevant* details to relay.

Be prepared to "have the answers" to anticipated questions. For instance, with our patient above with the diabetic ulcer, the wound specialist might ask about the patient's nutritional status. Nutrition plays a part in the body's ability to heal itself, so having that information available in case they ask for it makes sense. The worst interactions with doctors end up being the ones where they stump you. Have your notes available and try to pull up the patient's chart before dialing the doctor so you can quickly answer their questions. The best response if you don't have the right answers is "I can find out for you." With a little planning and experience, getting caught unprepared to answer the doctor's questions will become less common. When you are prepared for the conversation with the docs, you will sound more professional and they'll begin to trust and respect you for it. In time, they'll cut you some slack if you slip up once in a while.

Not every exchange with your colleagues will be cheerful and sometimes you'll have to deal with colorful personalities. Mind your manners if someone has an attitude or you disagree. Rather than arguing, try to see both sides by asking "Could you help me understand the advantage of this versus that?" You may cause the other person to think twice about what they've said and maybe they'll see your point of view. Some people you encounter will be having a bad day. They may seem miserable, grumpy, or just present with a bad attitude. Don't let the sass bring you down; you have no idea what that person went through earlier in the shift.

I'll never forget working in the ER and helping to treat a 1-year-old suffering from an asthma attack. We worked on that kiddo for hours with every treatment, but eventually, we had to intubate her. It took 40 minutes to stabilize her on a portable vent so she could be transported across the city to another hospital that had a pediatric ICU. The doctor I worked with did a phenomenal job and we felt good about what we were able to do for our tiny patient. A few hours later, we received word from the receiving hospital that the baby died shortly after arrival. We were completely devastated, but our doc still had 25 patients in the ER to treat.

I will tell you she was not a ray of sunshine for the remainder of the night. I caught some sideways glances and eye rolls from patients throughout the shift that had no idea what had happened earlier…they probably just thought our doc was being a jerk or had no bedside manner. I always remember that night and how difficult it was to rally and continue to work with our patients when we actually needed to just sit down somewhere and cry. Assume every attitude you encounter at work is because of something like what that ER doc went through and show empathy rather than firing back. The off-chance their bad mood truly was because of a tragedy, your kindness may go a long way for them.

Smile all day long as often as you can. Staying pleasant with the lab, the pharmacy, physical therapists, nutritionists, the respiratory therapists…it will all serve you well the day your patient needs something from one of them and looks to you for a small miracle. Keep positive vibes attached to your name and you should flourish in your new nursing career.

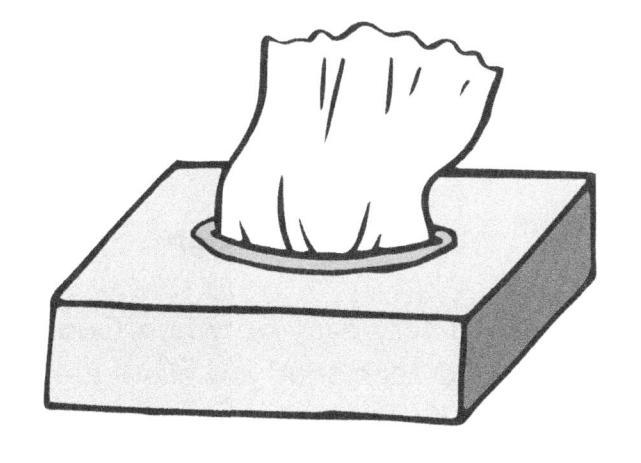

Handling the Emotions

Caught Up in Your Feels

Here it is, the real shit they don't teach you in nursing school. If you thought memorizing lab values, figuring out your ABGs, and pharmacology made nursing challenging, just wait until the world starts tugging on your heartstrings. You will witness miracles throughout your career as well as catastrophes. People will cry tears of joy, sadness, grief, and fear and you will be their rock. Among many other things, nursing is a profession with high emotional demand and you should be well aware of this from Day One.

It's Okay to Laugh

I learned very early on when I worked as an EMT and ED tech that you absolutely must learn to laugh if you are going to process what you will see and work with on a daily basis. Many in healthcare develop a dark sense of humor that would appall outsiders. Still, there will be times when you have no other choice but to laugh. One of those times was the night I met High-Five Freddie.

I was working as an Emergency Department Technician on the night shift during nursing school. A security guard from the waiting room yelled to the back that they needed a stretcher and some help out on the sidewalk. One of the nurses and I ran outside with a stretcher to find a beat-up Honda pulled halfway up the curb and a frantic couple yelling in Spanish beside it. They pointed to the backseat where we found an unconscious man who didn't appear to be breathing. Without wasting time, the nurse grabbed some legs and

I grabbed some arms and we hoisted the man out of the car and onto our stretcher.

The nurse jumped on top of the man, straddling him, and began chest compressions. I reached for the railings on the stretcher and locked them into place, then booked it through the doors to the ER. Racing through the hallway to our resuscitation room, the nurse continued CPR and I continued driving the stretcher like I stole it. Help had been summoned and we were met in the resus room by the whole ER team and doctor. We started cutting clothes, attaching monitors, ventilating, and looking for IV access.

Through the chaos, the doctor simply said, "Stop." We didn't, so he shouted, "Everyone STOP! Look at the patient." We stopped and observed. The man was blue and gray and still conformed to the position he was in while laid in the backseat of the old Honda. Most noticeable, his right hand was raised straight up in the air as if he was presenting for a high-five. Rigor had already set in and we didn't even notice. The doctor couldn't help but smirk. "I'm sorry to say, but I think High-Five Freddie here is gone. He's been gone for hours. Cover him up." He snapped his gloves off and walked away shaking his head.

Now, working in an emergency department it is common to deal with death and tragedy. So common that you must develop effective coping mechanisms or all of the negativity would debilitate you. I will tell you that, while we all agreed there was nothing funny about this patient's passing, there was humor in the way that we couldn't see on the dimly-lit sidewalk that this patient was beyond saving. The nurse took a bit of teasing for how enthusiastically he had jumped on top of the man while I was accused of nearly killing more people with my stretcher-driving skills than I would have saved. If you have respect for patients like High-Five Freddie in your heart, you can in good conscience laugh at the lighter side of situations.

It's Okay to Cry

Our vulnerable human qualities sometimes help to make us great nurses, as this line of work is not for the cold-hearted. We are all guaranteed to catch feelings at one point or another at work, but we owe it to our patients to remain human and remain connected to them. Dealing with tragedy, death, and grief are things for which we will build coping mechanisms. With experience, time, and communication with our friends, families, and colleagues, we will practice dealing with grief and we *will* get better at responding in healthy ways. But we must not, for our patients' sakes, become callous. When a grieving family member locks eyes with us, they will need to see validation for their own emotions in *our* eyes, not indifference.

I recall one of the most emotional moments I have had during a shift. I was caring for an end-of-life patient who was waiting for transport to a hospice facility. He had completely stopped eating several days prior and his breathing patterns indicated he didn't have much time left. COVID had limited our visitor policy so I had to make arrangements with our nursing supervisor to allow his family members to come up all at once to see him.

The patient's daughter and two granddaughters entered the room as I was situating his pillows and blankets. Tears welled up immediately in their eyes as they started softly asking questions. I explained he did not have much time and they should take the opportunity to talk to him. I remained in the room, silent and supportive, as the family whispered that everything would be okay to the patient and brushed through his hair with their hands. All at once, it seemed, we noticed his chest had stopped rising. In a second, three sets of eyes were looking right at me to read my response. I froze. From the hallway, I could hear the telemetry monitor dinging away, but my charge nurse who was aware of the situation quickly silenced the alarm.

I tried to speak but my words were caught in my throat. I flashed back through my own experiences losing loved ones and I knew that if I opened my mouth to say anything at all, that rush of emotions would wash over me and I'd completely lose my composure. I had seen death on the job plenty of times before, but something about this scene was just different, and goddamn was it sad.

My charge nurse Virginia became my hero that day. She entered the room and took the daughter by her hands. In a soft, caring voice, she said, "He's leaving us now. Would you like to pray with me?" There were nods and tears as Virginia joined hands with the family and they prayed. Afterward, she said a few more soothing words, then opened the window in the room a few inches so the patient's spirit was free to go. I was in awe.

I have thought back on that afternoon a thousand times and, each time, I am grateful for having been through that experience.

Virginia is a veteran nurse who knew exactly what to say and do to handle the situation while she also knew exactly how to remain human and offer herself to the family. Always remember that in the event your patient passes away with their family present, each member of his or her family now becomes your patient. You should offer yourself to them, ensure they are both safe and comfortable, and provide support to them during this time.

    About a year after that patient passed away, I was presented with an almost identical situation. This time, I was precepting an orientee and was covering another nurse while she went on a lunch break. One of that nurse's patients was being cared for with comfort measures only after her condition had quickly deteriorated over just a few days. Her husband was at her bedside when the familiar ding ding on the telemetry monitor prompted us to respond to her room.

    I saw the husband holding her hand and looking up at us, holding back tears and staying strong for his wife as she slipped away. With a deep breath, I shut my eyes and played back the scene once again of Virginia consoling that family. I approached with a soft voice, placed my hand on the husband's shoulder, and explained that his wife was leaving us. I told him to speak to her as she could still hear him and that we would not leave his side. We stood, my orientee and myself, with our hands clasped in front of us and our heads down in silence. The woman took her last breath, her husband whimpered softly at her side, and I opened the window.

The sad days are hard, but they get easier as you learn to process them. The patient's husband took his time in the room with his wife. He eventually came out into the hallway and found me to shake my hand. I asked if he was okay to drive, he said he was, and he gave me a tight hug. He simply said, "Thank you." We have the opportunity as nurses to ensure families don't face loss alone, to provide sympathy as well as services or support they may need, and to keep them safe while they grieve. Also, it's okay to cry with them.

It's Okay to be Afraid

In March of 2020, COVID19 was raging across the globe and, shortly after it reached pandemic status, we received word at my hospital that we were to begin receiving and treating COVID patients. We didn't have much time to prepare, so a team of our facilities personnel armed with plywood, jigsaws, and a 5 lb hand sledge started knocking out windows on our cardiac interventional unit to retrofit HEPA filtration units to the rooms.

    In the first few months of treating patients, two members of our staff contracted COVID and died. Several more of our staff members inadvertently carried the virus home with them where it infected their family members and more lives were lost. Marissa, whose unit had drawn the short straw and became the COVID unit, was working with and caring for infected patients each and every day. Staff dwindled and, before long, every nurse in the hospital was being pulled to the COVID unit to work shifts on a weekly (or more) basis.

    The work was grueling as we entered springtime. The HEPA units removed any air conditioning from the patient rooms and, under the layers of Tyvek, gloves, gowns, and caps, we were drenched in sweat. We blistered and bled from behind our ears and the bridges of our noses where N95 masks rubbed us raw. I recall working nearly an entire 12-hour shift without water because I wasn't able or willing to remove my mask to drink. Once home, Marissa and I had set up our own make-shift decontamination station in the garage consisting of bleach wipes, Lysol spray, and homemade hand sanitizer (because every store was sold out). Getting undressed in the garage and cleaning off before running upstairs to shower added another 30 minutes to each workday. Worst of all, through all the blood, sweat, and tears, patients were not getting better.

It was terrifying to go to work and risk exposure to yourself and your family. Just as scary was building relationships with your patients as you would spend weeks caring for them but no treatments seem to work. People got sicker and sicker, slowly being starved of oxygen. Marissa held many hands and played music for her patients as they came to terms with the grim reality of their situation. If she entered the room with an iPad, it was as if she was handing the patient a death sentence. See, the hospital's iPad was signed out from the security room so the patient could video chat with his or her family one last time before being intubated. Once placed on a vent, few patients would ever breathe on their own again and most would be switched off after just a few days.

The fear during the pandemic was constant. Each time things would seem as though they were improving, we would get another wave of COVID patients and some would not survive. We hadn't seen our families in months and couldn't bear to go on social media which was loaded with anti-mask protests and conspiracy theorists. Finally, after nearly a year, our treatments began to work. Antiviral medications, convalescent plasma, and strong steroids were turning patients around better than anything we had tried before. One morning, our entire staff lined the hallway outside of our COVID unit as our first patient had fought her way off the ventilator, out of the ICU, and right out our front door. We cheered and she cried, grateful to be alive.

There will be downright terrifying moments during your career as a nurse. I have been deposed following a patient's death to determine if I had responsibility or could have done anything differently. I have fought as hard as I could to keep someone alive despite the universe having other plans. I have drawn shades and moved patients' beds away from windows during a tornado warning. There will be fear, but you are not alone. It is fear shared by all of your coworkers and all 28 million nurses across the world. It is okay to be afraid, but it is necessary to work through that fear to keep our patients safe. Remember! Not everyone is strong or courageous enough to be a nurse. But you are.

It's Okay to be Proud

One emotion that we don't always talk about and isn't so obvious with regards to nursing is pride. Pride sometimes carries negative connotations or can be misassociated with hubris. The great, late comedian George Carlin once said, "I could never understand ethnic or national pride, 'cause to me, pride should be reserved for something you achieve or attain on your own, not something that happens by accident of birth." By his logic, I shouldn't be *proud* to have been born English and German through no control of my own. I was born in New Jersey, but I didn't control that so I shouldn't be a "proud" New Jerseyan. Rather, I should be proud of my achievements…things in my life I have worked hard for. My nursing license is one of those things.

Why should we be *proud* to be nurses? Can't anyone just go to nursing school and become a nurse? Despite nursing being one of the most popular professions in the world, not everyone is cut out to be a nurse. Some never make it past the bodily fluids and the smells.

Others can't handle the stress or the workload. A T-chart weighing the pros and cons of becoming a nurse may look very different if made by a nurse versus anyone else. That is because nursing means working long shifts, holidays, overnights, being cursed at, hit, bit, and clawed. It means exposure to infectious disease, witnessing death, abuse, and tragedy. It means a commitment to life-long learning, working in an ever-changing environment with technology that evolves every single year. With so many challenges, how could we be proud to be nurses?

    My answer is simple. Because we can handle it. Someone has to be there for the sick, the troubled, and the injured. Someone has to be there for the beginning and end of life. Someone has to be there willing to save lives, accept the successes and the failures, and do it all within the stringent guidelines of the policies, protocols, and best nursing practice. We laugh, we cry, and sometimes we are downright terrified. A nurse's worst shift doesn't come close to someone else's worst shift. But we are strong enough to handle it and have a duty to protect our patients.

    I am a proud nurse because I have personally saved lives. Had I not become a nurse, there is a good likelihood that someone in my place would have done the same, but there is no certainty. During one of my first nursing shifts, I was fresh out of our hospital's EKG training class. I was looking over the telemetry monitor on our unit when I spotted an odd-looking rhythm. I printed a strip and started to measure as I had been taught. Slow heart rate, about 40 bpm, with regular QRS complexes. The P waves were there too, regular, but they didn't seem to coalesce with the QRS. Was this a third-degree heart block? If so, the patient was in serious trouble.

    I brought the strip to my charge nurse and was told that it was a stable type 2 block and the treatment team was aware. I argued that the rhythm was much worse and pointed out my concerns on the little strip of thermal paper. When my charge nurse wasn't convinced, I went to the nurse caring for that patient who agreed with the charge. The patient, a woman in her 30's, was fatigued but otherwise alert and felt fine. I tracked down my preceptor, showed her the strip, and pressed on that this was a potentially-lethal 3rd-degree block. She pursed her lips, made a few measurements of her own on some freshly-printed strips, and picked up the phone. Within minutes, the electrophysiology team was rushing the patient out of her room for an emergent pacemaker. My preceptor offered me a high-five and told me, "Good save."

I have saved other people as well. I did abdominal thrusts on a patient choking on a potato. Embarrassed, she turned to me with a scowl and asked if I would handle my grandmother that way. "Yes ma'am, if she was choking on a roasted potato, I certainly would." I have performed CPR on patients both in the field as an EMT and in the hospital setting who have survived cardiac arrest. During my time in the emergency department, I spotted a psych patient slouched in a chair who just didn't look right. To be honest, she looked like that creepy girl who crawled out of the well in The Ring. When I called out to her she didn't respond. I shook her shoulder and she tensed up. When I moved her hair out of the way I saw a blue face, bulging eyes, and a swollen tongue. Wrapped tightly around her neck was about 6 feet of gauze which she had removed from a self-inflicted wound on her arm. With the help of another ED tech, we wrestled her to the stretcher and were able to cut away the gauze, reopening her airway, without causing her any further injury.

Nursing allowed me to be there for these patients and others in their time of need. I'm proud to have completed nursing school, the toughest academic pursuit of my life, proud to have been a successful EMT, ED tech, and now a nurse. I am proud that nurses I have oriented have become successful as well. I am proud of the way I have learned to handle some of the toughest situations in life and that my presence has made a difference to other people when they are in their darkest hours. I do not see nursing pride as having a downside; rather I believe you can be proud *to be* proud of all you have achieved getting this far, plus for all the challenges coming your way in your career that you accept and are prepared for.

It's Okay to Feel

Few professions are as emotionally, physically, and mentally taxing as nursing. As a nurse, you will see the beginning of life as well as the end of it. You'll be given the opportunity to be there for others during miracles and tragedies. Those events will stick with you and you will always remember how they made you feel. I remember how I felt when I heard the blood-curdling screams of a mother as her 6-year-old daughter was whisked away by child protective services for suspected sexual abuse. I remember the joy and uncontrolled laughter when a liver patient who, after he had been told he would not survive the night, got the news that a new liver was in the air on its way to the hospital for him, and the transplant team was scrubbing in. I laughed along with him, I have cried along with others, and I've learned it is okay to have feelings in this line of work.

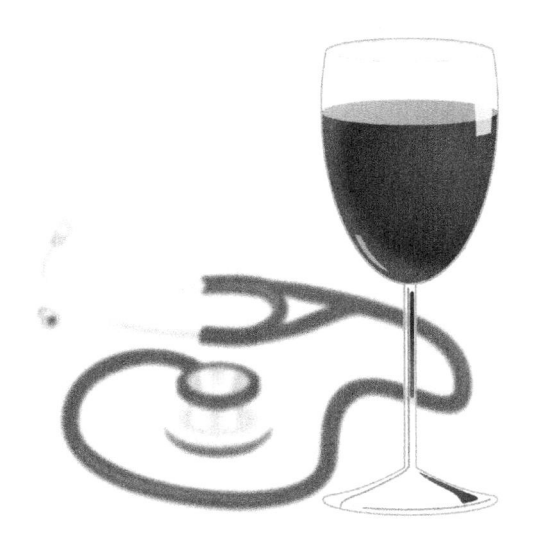

Conclusion

A Sigh of Relief and a Nice Ride Home

You never thought you'd make it, but you've just completed your very first nursing shift. Chances are your brain is firing from synapses you didn't know you had. Your back, legs, and feet may be sore and you might have had to adjust your rear-view mirror before heading home because you are simply too tired to sit up straight. But you did it. By now, you have already leaped over so many hurdles and your next shift will be so much easier because of it. You've found the bathrooms, learned where the code cart is and how to call for help, and you met your preceptor. With pages full of notes, you still have plenty of learning to do, but now you feel more prepared to fine-tune that learning and become an expert on your unit. Best of all, you were met with more smiling faces than you were prepared for and it seems as though you'll be getting along with your new colleagues just fine.

      Tomorrow will be easier, but you know you will face challenges at every stage of your career. Nursing is not easy and it's not for the weak. But you aren't lazy and you are strong as hell, so you are not worried about it. Before pulling out of the parking lot, you check your phone. Maybe it's loaded with text messages from family members who can't wait to hear about your first day. Maybe it's just your background photo of your goldfish Sheldon. Either way, your day is over and it's time to head home and hit the shower. Enjoy your dinner, your glass of wine, and take some time to rest up. On behalf of your preceptor, your managers, your fellow nurses, and your coworkers, it was great working with you today.

      Here are some final thoughts as you continue through your orientation period. You will learn, practice your skills, and get better every shift. Nursing is HARD. But you can do it. As a matter of fact, thank God you are here to do it. Because if it wasn't for you being there for your patients, looking out for them, advocating for them, making them feel safe, and getting them better...who knows what would happen. They need you, so keep your chin up when things get tough.

    Keep nurse friends to help you get through the day-to-day. My best friend is a nurse. I married her. Only nurses know what other nurses go through, so it's nice to have someone on speed dial who you can vent to and who will understand your troubles. They'll also celebrate your victories with you. Grow together in the profession and have each other's backs...you'll be glad you did. Nursing affords a comfortable lifestyle, allowing us to *work to live* rather than living to work. Many full-time nurses are off four or more days out of the week and can spend that time with their families, doing their favorite hobbies, or just taking in the joys life has to offer. Few professions provide you the opportunity to make a positive impact on people's lives the way nursing does. Stay humble, appreciate the opportunity, and be prepared to work hard.

MEET THE CONTRIBUTORS

Here are the incredible nurses who provided advice, tips, and insight to make this book possible.

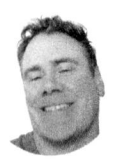

William R. Case, RN: Bill became a nurse after a long and successful teaching career. He now brings his skills in teaching and organization into the healthcare setting. His calm nature and warm personality make him a favorite among his patients.

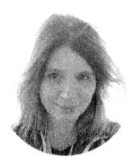

Michelle Clark, RN: Michelle is a charge nurse with a passion for caring. The quintessential team player, Michelle is a natural leader who advocates for her patients and new nurses alike.

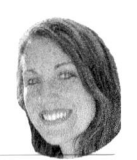

Gabrielle Corbin, PCT: Gabby is the tech you'd want to face the craziest shifts with. Smart, quick, and cool under pressure, she has your back. Gabby is completing courses to become an ultrasound technician.

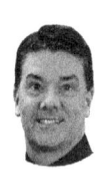

John Davis, RN: John is a telemetry charge nurse on a specialized cardiac unit with nearly 3 decades of experience. He makes strong connections with his patients, colleagues, and the brand new nurses who he welcomes to the hospital.

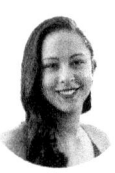

Marissa Dovell, RN: Marissa is a critical care nurse working in trauma/medical. An expert in patient assessment, efficiency, and getting those tough IVs, she earned awards both for her efforts as a preceptor and her patient care.

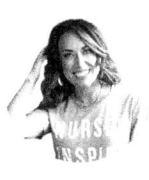

Cat Golden, BSN, RN: Cat worked for nearly a decade as a pediatric nurse when she realized nurses needed a new level of support. She founded Nurses Inspire Nurses and, through community, merch, events and an endless amount of fun has grown to attract national media attention including a feature in Forbes and an appearance on the Kelly Clarkson Show.

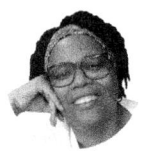

Wanda Goodmond, MSN, RN: Wanda is a beacon of wisdom for nurses of any experience level. With over 20 years of experience, Wanda works with a cool head, provides a voice for patients and fellow nurses, and has a wealth of knowledge on everything from reading ECGs to medications and procedures.

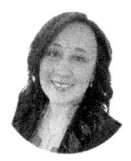

Michelle Lasota, BSN, RN, CHPN: Michelle is an oncology nurse who spent much of her career working in hospice care. Her caring and compassion are unmatched and drew the attention of filmmakers who created a documentary about her, *The Nurse with the Purple Hair*.

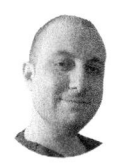

Raymond Lawton, RN: Ray's multitasking abilities lent themselves well to his work in long-term subacute care. He now works in the acute care setting with EP, vascular, and cardiology patients.

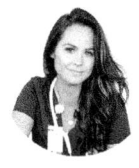

Tori Meskin, BSN RNC-NIC: Tori is an esteemed NICU nurse, successful blogger, and co-host of The Cellfie Show, a medical podcast where she speaks on healthcare, self-care, and the down and dirty in between.

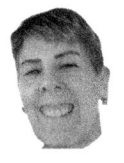

Patty Stark, RN: Patty is a veteran critical care nurse with over 40 years of experience. She currently works as an Assistant Nurse Manager for a cardiac surgical intensive care unit.

71 QUICK & AWESOME NURSING TIPS

1. Carry liquid bandage with you to work for those pesky knicks and cuts on your hands. They can easily get infected and bandaids won't survive your frequent hand-washing and glove-wearing.

2. Double glove when dealing with a messy situation. After cleaning up the bulk of the mess, remove the layer of soiled gloves to reveal clean ones which won't just spread the filthiness around as you finish up.

3. IV pump buzzing in a super chatty patient's room? Give another nurse or your unit coordinator a call on your handheld phone so you can chat about very important nursing stuff while situating the IV pump. A quick thumbs up to your patient and off you go!

4. Solidifier in an ice bag turns melted ice into the same sort of frozen jelly round in reusable ice packs. It lasts longer and prevents leaking!

5. To make an amazing warm compress, wet a towel with hot water, then wrap up in a chuck with the smooth side against the towel, soft side toward the patient. A bit of tape to secure it all and you have a compress that will last longer and keep your patient dry.

6. To keep the bell of your stethoscope clean while assessing a bloody or otherwise soiled patient, simply cover the bell with a clean glove.

7. Your stethoscope can be used as a hearing aid if your nearly-deaf patient can't understand you. Place the stethoscope in his ears and speak softly into the bell, getting a bit closer until he can hear you.

8. If a patient knows you are counting respirations, he may become conscious of his breathing pattern. Instead, continue to hold a radial pulse and pretend to count the beats, looking past the wrist to the patient's rising chest.

9. Vicks is your friend for all sorts of stinkiness. A bit of Vicks on your mustache area or rubbed into your

mask can cut through the worst GI bleed smells.

10. Soaking a length of roll gauze with mouthwash and hanging it in the corner of a patient room can act as a diffuser and help cover up stinkiness.

11. When you need to transfuse fluids quickly and a pressure bag isn't handy, grab the trusty manual blood pressure cuff. Wrap the cuff around the IV bag and inflate to squeeze. As the bag empties, pump the cuff a few more times to keep it tight.

12. Make your own badge buddies! Write your info on an index card, cut it to size, and laminating or wrapping in clear tape is a great way to keep important-to-remember information like phone numbers, names, and pin codes available and at your fingertips.

13. If you are having trouble adjusting to military time at work, set your cell phone to only display military time! After a few weeks, you'll master the change and could probably switch your phone back to a 12-hour format.

14. Don't make a habit of working through your lunch break, especially if you are working 12-hour shifts. You are entitled to your breaks and it's on your facility to make sure you are covered for them.

15. When communicating with your patient, get down on their level. When a patient is in bed and you are standing, you may present yourself as authoritative rather than caring and compassionate. Stoop, squat, or pull up a chair so you can look your patient right in the eyes as you speak and listen.

16. If you can't find a good spot to place an IV in a patient, try wrapping the arm with a warm compress and letting it dangle off the bed for a few minutes.

17. If your patient's veins keep blowing out when attempting to place an IV, try this: the moment you puncture the vein, immediately release the tourniquet. This will reduce pressure in the vein as you advance the angiocath and it will be less likely to blow.

18. Always bring your water bottle with you when you document. By making

this a habit, you can ensure you stay hydrated even during the busiest shifts.

19. If there are skills or subjects that trip you up during your orientation, make a list of goals for each of them and share the list with your preceptor. This will help you to master these areas while helping your preceptor to better understand what to focus on.

20. Don't be reactive if someone has a bad attitude toward you. Rather, stay professional and give it a bit of time. People who work in hospitals encounter emotional distress at some point and commonly lash out at others. Better to take the high road and, most of the time, you'll end up with an apology rather than an enemy.

21. Get your own liability insurance. Hospitals will cover you when it suits them but will also throw you under the bus if it doesn't.

22. Listen to veteran nurses as they explain procedures to patients, perform admissions, and provide discharge teaching. No sense in trying to

reinvent the wheel, so I emulate many of the best nurses I work with when I teach my patients.

23. In a code or emergency, if you need multiple jobs done at once, assign them to people in the room rather than just shouting them all out. This is most efficient and will ensure each person knows what she is doing.

24. Use your paid time off! Do your best to work a schedule that won't cause burnout and, if you *do* start to feel exhausted all the time, give yourself a nice chunk of time off.

25. Always flush a patient's IV before he or she leaves your unit for a procedure. It may have flushed well when you assessed it, but double-checking ensures the procedure won't be delayed to obtain IV new access if there are issues.

26. Trust your coworkers, but don't always take their word for things. If a CNA tells you they prepped your patient for the OR, that's great but YOU are still the nurse. The only way to know for sure is with your eyeballs, so go check.

27. Don't be miserable at your job. If you are unhappy working on your unit for whatever reason, start looking for a change of scenery immediately. There is no sense in letting your job bring you down, especially when there are so many opportunities out there for a change.

28. When you have more than two things to get done, write each task down in a list, then go back over the list and number the tasks in order of priority.

29. Don't answer "doctor" questions. There is no mistake, nurses are extremely knowledgeable and great resources to patients looking for information. By "doctor questions," I'm talking about specifics regarding procedures, plans, and anything you may *think* you know but wouldn't bet your car on. Rather than guessing, save your breath and your time and arrange for the doctor to speak with the patient or family member.

30. Ask if you can visit other units or, even better, procedure areas. You can do this either before, after, or during your shift depending on how busy things

are. It is invaluable to see other departments, how they operate, and to watch with your own eyes the procedures you have been teaching your patients about.

31. Use a report sheet as a guide. A report sheet will prompt you to ask about missing details when, at the end of giving a report, the other nurse asks you "Any questions?" Rather than trying to recall what may be missing, you would be staring at a report sheet with blank spaces waiting to be filled in.

32. In a Code Blue, take the time to prepare the room. Once two nurses are focused on providing CPR, everyone else should quickly empty the room of unnecessary furniture and equipment and pull the bed away from the wall to allow for intubation. This takes only seconds but is much more difficult if you wait for the code team to arrive.

33. Ask a patient to turn away from you and cough the moment you give them an injection. I use this trick when administering subcutaneous heparin

and, many times, it tricks the patient's brain so he won't feel the needle at all.

34. Expect to lose pens, so always have plenty of them.

35. A patient talking your ear off when you have a lot of work left to do? This takes some acting, but I will look toward an imaginary person in the doorway and put up a "wait a minute" finger. I will look concerned, say something like "Is it bed 12 again?" then turn back to my patient apologizing before quickly leaving the room. Desperate times call for desperate measures.

36. Document defensively. This means you should write notes to cover your ass in case a patient were to ever sue you. In school, I was taught to document by exception; this is not always the best way. "Pertinent negatives" have their place in your nursing notes. Find a patient sitting on the floor? "Pt found AAOx4 sitting comfortably on floor with no distress. Pt reports sitting on floor because bed was 'uncomfortable.' Pt denies falling, striking head or back, or any other injury/complaint."

37. Get to work a few minutes early. This is for your benefit and no one else's. There is a big difference between rushing out of your coat and into report versus taking your time to sip some coffee, review the assignment board, and take a peek at your patients before officially starting your shift.

38. When you are in report, make a habit of checking certain parts of each patient's chart before moving on so you can ask questions if anything seems off or is confusing. I always look at the medication list, IV infusions, most recent labs, and the last physician note outlining the updated plan of care.

39. If there is an emergency in your patient's room, yell for help as loud as you can and include the room number. When seconds count, shouting "I need help in Room 8!" can save your colleagues valuable seconds.

40. Set up your report sheet in a way that you can read through it easily when handing off to another nurse. Lead with the patient demographics, then

discuss history, follow it with current status and labs, assessment, and end with plan-of-care. This will keep you from jumping around when giving report and reduces any confusion or missed information.

41. Pay attention to how much your patients pee. It sounds odd but low urine output is a huge indicator that your patient is not doing well. Less than 30 mL per hour? Check how much fluid your patient is drinking or receiving intravenously and consider calling the doc.

42. Never, ever grab a bottle of peri cleaner or barrier ointment bare-handed. Those items get grabbed and used while wiping butts and are usually filthy.

43. Don't watch medical shows with non-medical field family or friends. You WILL drive them nuts as you critique the authenticity of the information, question why it takes 3 attending doctors to perform a CT scan, or burst out laughing when the paramedics slam through the ER doors shouting at everyone.

44. Burp your IV bags. After spiking your bag of fluids and before squeezing the drip chamber, turn your bag upside down and squeeze the air out of the bag. This will prevent air from running into your tubing when the fluids run out and you can simply repeat the process for your next bag. This saves you from having to prime the tubing again!

45. Protect your patients' IVs! Assume your patient's sole purpose in life is to get their tubing caught on something and yank out that beautifully and painstakingly placed IV. Extra tape, netting, even bandage materials can all help to protect the IV…don't skip this step.

46. Verbalize safety. I always make a point of explaining safety actions I take to my patient and anyone else in the room as I perform them. Things like removing clutter from the floor, turning on a bed alarm, or hand-washing can be said out loud. Doing so helps to maintain a safety culture and reassures those around you that you are a safe nurse.

47. Homemade shoe spray. Your work shoes may get a bit stinky, especially after working several long shifts in a row. An effective and inexpensive solution is mixing rubbing alcohol with water in a spray bottle and lightly misting the shoes inside and out. The alcohol will sanitize the shoes, killing the bacteria that cause odor.

48. Make sure your name is on your stethoscope! Protect your investment! Hopefully no one intentionally tries to steal from you, but most stethoscopes look the same and we call tend to carry the same types or brands. Engraving is nice but Sharpie is better than nothing.

49. Manage your patient's expectations. If you are too busy to stop moving but your patient asks for something like a comfort item, don't promise to come right back with one. Chances are, your patient is *not* busy and has nothing to do but sit and wait for you. Be honest about the likelihood you will return in a given timeframe or simply tell them you will be back as soon as possible.

50. Whenever I gather equipment and supplies for a procedure like a Foley placement or a dressing change, I like to collect everything I need in a basin. I toss a few extras of everything in there so I rarely have to leave the patient's room in the middle of the job. I find it easier to have extras and return them all afterward than to go scrambling for something in the middle of a procedure.

51. It can get exhausting when a patient has several family members who call or ask for updates throughout the shift. Do your best to appoint one family member as the "family representative." I do this VERY matter-of-factly. "We typically appoint one person as the family rep. It helps keep the information and updates streamlined and gives us more time to focus on caring for your loved one."

52. Make a to-do list for your nighttime on-call doctor. Overnight docs are often working a 24-hour shift and each phone call they receive takes away from their opportunity to rest. By creating a small list of things you need

such as PRN medication orders for all of your patients, you can make things easier for this doc while ensuring your patients are adequately cared for.

53. Stay in touch with your classmates from nursing school. Reach out to them frequently to find out where they have landed jobs and if they enjoy their workplaces. This is the beginning of your professional network and could lead to wonderful opportunities in the future.

54. Ask where you can find your facility's protocols (most hospitals have an online database) and print out the most frequently used. Writing a condensed version of the protocol on a 3x5 card and keeping them handy is a great way to ensure you react to situations such as sepsis, hypoglycemia, or blood transfusions appropriately.

55. Listen in when doctors speak to your patient. Not only is it a great way to learn, but you can also help your patients if they don't recall all of the education or instructions provided during the conversation.

56. Learn the equipment and tasks within your scope of practice, even if they are normally done by someone else. Phlebotomy, ECGs, and skin prep for procedures aren't usually done by nurses where I work. You should still learn how to perform these tasks in the event the unit is short-staffed or there is an emergency and a phlebotomist or technician isn't around.

57. Always know the "why" behind each medication you are giving. This is useful in keeping your patient safe and monitoring associated labs and vital signs. Plus, if your patient asks you why you are giving them the med, "because the doctor told me to" is not a professional answer.

58. Believe family members when they tell you something is wrong. They know the patient much better than you do.

59. Believe the patient when they say something is wrong. Every patient that has looked me in the eyes and told me they were going to die ended up either dying or coming pretty damn close.

60. Confirm pulses with a doppler if you can't feel them. I lost a patient who was transferred to me from another hospital with critical limb ischemia to his leg. By the time that hospital realized his leg was in trouble, it was too late. An aggressive intervention was necessary and the patient died on the table. If you don't feel a pulse in a lower extremity, confirm it. If you still don't get a pulse, call the doctor immediately.

61. If you have a few minutes at the end of your shift, review your patients' charts and physician notes so you can provide an updated plan of care to the next nurse. This is an important step to make sure everyone on the care team knows what is next for the patient.

62. If you write out a brief report on your patients for the nurse covering your lunch break, ask for that paper back to hand off to your charge nurse at the end of shift. Oftentimes the charge nurse will need the same synopsis for each patient on the unit and using the same report slip saves time.

63. Cluster care, especially with isolation patients. If you have the means to call into the room prior to entering, do this and find out if the patient needs anything. So long as medications and other orders aren't particularly time-sensitive, collect everything you will need and go into the patient's room once to give meds, assess, and provide care and hygiene.

64. As the new nurse at your job, you may have ideas to improve something. This could be a change in the charting software, recommending a new piece of equipment to keep patients safer, or a new method of communication. Write these ideas down and, a bit later when you are more established, run them by your manager. We should never stop trying to improve our hospitals and the care of our patients.

65. Keep your eyes out for mentors at your workplace. While much of your attention will be on your preceptor in your first few weeks, pay attention to the nurses that seem to have it all together or provide the best care.

66. Placing IVs intimidates many new nurses and is sometimes challenging even for veteran nurses. Practice makes perfect, so ask around if any patients will need a new IV. You'll be doing yourself and your colleagues a favor the more IVs you place on your unit.

67. With patient assessment, always "see it with your own eyes." Don't trust what you heard in report or read in the patient's chart. Many times, I have reviewed assessment data that was completely false or had changed.

68. Always ensure you have good IV access on your patient at the start and throughout your shift. If an IV looks like trouble, is leaking, or doesn't have a good rate of flow, consider replacing it ASAP rather than waiting for it to blow or infiltrate.

69. At the start of your shift, sanitize your workstation, phone, and anything else you'll be touching a lot throughout the day. At the end of the shift, sanitize your pens, cellphone, name badge, water bottle, and all of the other

equipment that you bring home or to the car.

70. Find a good quiet place where you can take a 30-second break to chill out if you feel angry, overwhelmed, or stressed. This can be the med room, the supply closet…even a bathroom. Don't hesitate to take those 30 seconds to regroup and refocus.

71. Don't ever feel trapped in a job. If the bad shifts outweigh the good and you begin to dread each time you walk through the doors and clock in, it's time to shop around. Nursing offers a huge variety of careers and you will undoubtedly find the perfect match for you.

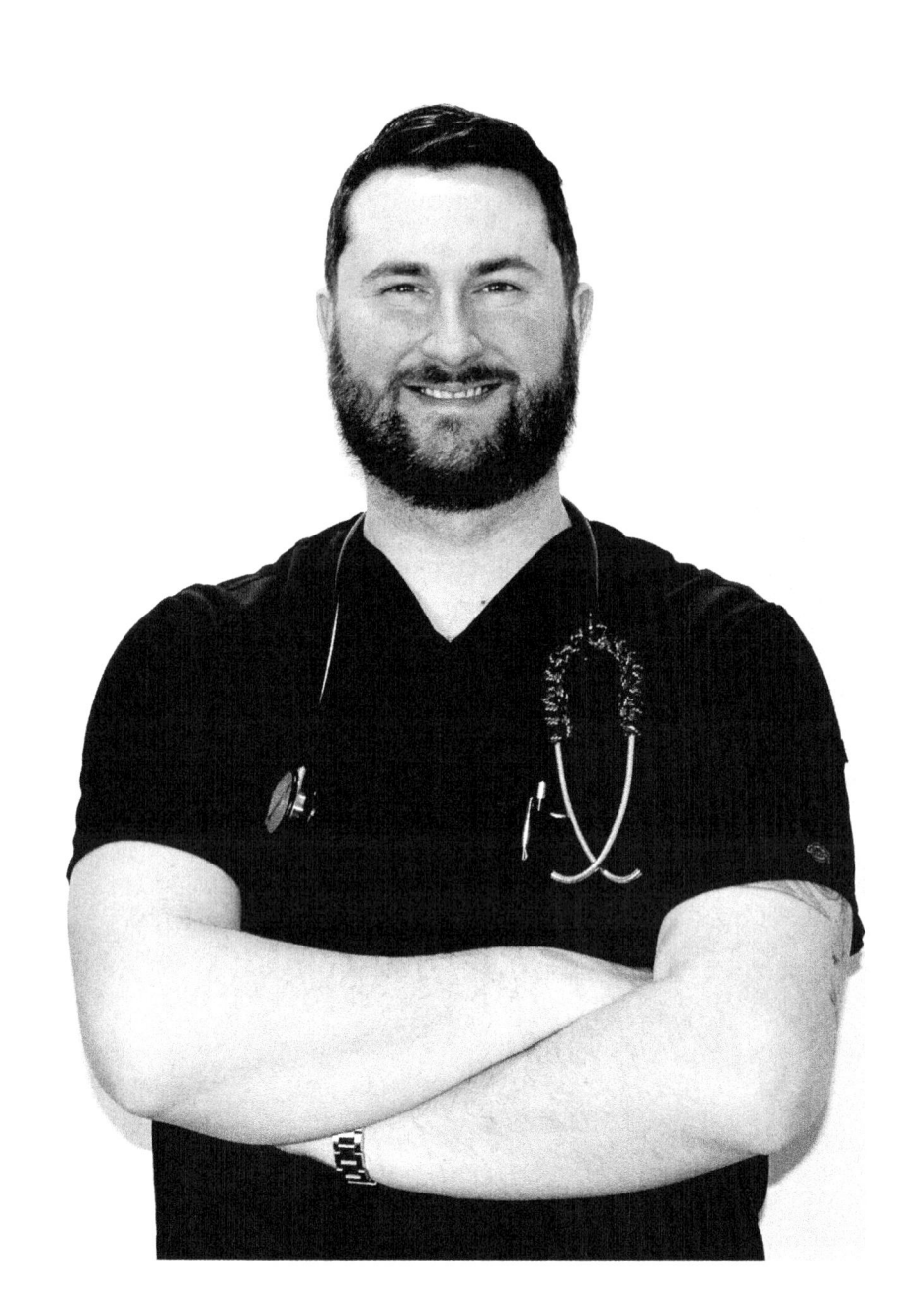

ABOUT THE AUTHOR

Dave Dovell, RN is a nurse, EMT, husband, and father. Since earning his Bachelor's degree in History from Rutgers University, Dave has worked a variety of jobs in education, restaurants, and management. Shortly after losing his best friend to leukemia, Dave was inspired to become a nurse. He quickly completed his nursing program (where he met his beautiful wife, Marissa) while working nights as an emergency department technician in Camden, NJ where he earned the Guardian Angel Award.

Dave works as an RN on a cardiac-stepdown unit where he was presented with the hospital's Star of the Month Award and has precepted several new nurses along the way. In addition to his work at the hospital, Dave is actively involved with a fast-growing cancer nonprofit in Philadelphia called Legacy of Hope, operates and writes for his blog, theNewRN.com, and freelances as a website designer for small businesses.

Most important to Dave are his family and close friends. Dave, Marissa, and their son Noah love going for hikes, trips to the aquarium, and taking day trips all over New Jersey. When they stay home, Dave enjoys playing guitar, trying new recipes in the kitchen, and spending time outside with an ice-cold beer.